ANYTHING BUT ORDINARY

UNUSUAL MEDICINE

BY JOHN MICKLOS, JR.

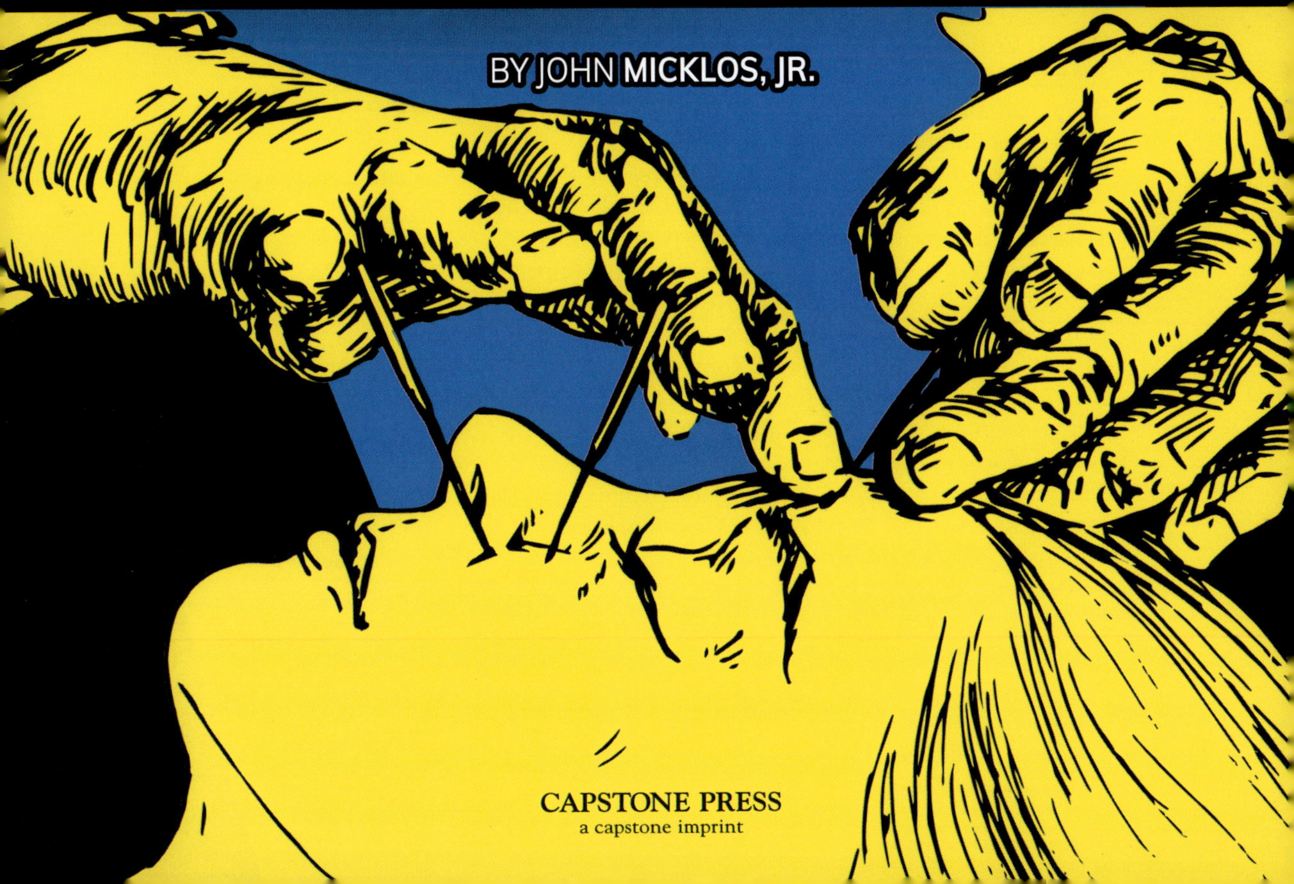

CAPSTONE PRESS
a capstone imprint

Capstone Captivate is published by Capstone Press,
an imprint of Capstone.
1710 Roe Crest Drive
North Mankato, Minnesota 56003
www.capstonepub.com

Library of Congress Cataloging-in-Publication data is available on the Library of Congress website.
ISBN 978-1-4966-8462-2 (library binding)
ISBN 978-1-4966-8482-0 (eBook PDF)

Editorial Credits

Editor: Mandy Robbins; Designer: Kyle Grenz; Media Researcher: Kelly Garvin; Production Specialist: Kathy McColley

Photo Credits

Alamy: The Natural HIstory Museum, 17; Getty Images: Bettmann, 13, picture alliance, 22, 39, Win McNamee/Staff, 41; iStockphoto: HRAUN, top 5; Newscom: AA/ABACA, 15, Abbas Idrees/Pacific Press, 23, Stewart Cook/Mirrorpix, 37; Science Source: BIOPHOTO Associates, 19, Frans Lanting/MINT Images, 25, R. Umesh Chandran, TDR, WHO, 11, Wellcome Images, 21; Shutterstock: Andrew Shapor, (scorpion) 35, argus, (sparks) design element, Artur Balytskyi, (viper) 35, Asakura1102, (water) 5, AshTproductions, 43, BarbaraDiniz, (spider) 35, basel101658, (dog) 29, Bjoern Wylezich, 30, Black creator 24, right 16, Bodar Tivadar, (fish) 35, Bokica, left 16, Cristina Romero Palma, bottom 34, Eroshka, (frog) 35, fivespots, top 34, frank60, 45, Golden Shrimp, (snake) 35, GzP_Design, (vessel) 5, igor malovic, (boy) 29, Jacky Co, (building) 29, Leremy, (peoples) 29, Lifeking, (nerve) 5, Maks TRV, (skeleton) 5, Malikov Aleksandr, 7, manusapon kasosod, 28, MarinaGrigorivna, right Cover, Martial Red, (germs) 29, Morphart Creation, middle Cover, ONYXprj, (organs) 5, P.S.Art-Design-Studio, 1, Panda Vector, (muscle) 5, (bw spider) 35, Performance Portraits, 27, Rvector, (phobia) 29, S.Jeshurun Vineeth Roshan, left Cover, Scharfsinn, 8, Schira, 10, Shidlovski, 33, Sketchi, (bottle) 35, stasia_ch, (octopus) 35, supanut piyakanont, (people) 29, Supawadee56, 31, tb-photography, 32, The Fisherman, (jellyfish) 35, vinap, (snake) 35, Yaroslav Shkuro, middle 16

Printed and bound in the USA.
PA117

TABLE OF CONTENTS

Words in **bold** are in the glossary.

The Wild World of Medicine

Most of the time, human bodies work well. But sometimes interesting and uncommon things happen. What if you had a 20-foot (6-meter) **tapeworm** living inside you? What if your legs swelled to become thick and painful? These things really happen to people.

When something goes wrong with our bodies, we often can trust doctors to fix it. Some treatments are simple. Others are more complicated or really surprising. What would you think about having leeches keep your wound clean? Did you know that sticking needles in your body can relieve pain, and sometimes laughter really is the best medicine? Check out some fascinating medical conditions and equally interesting treatments!

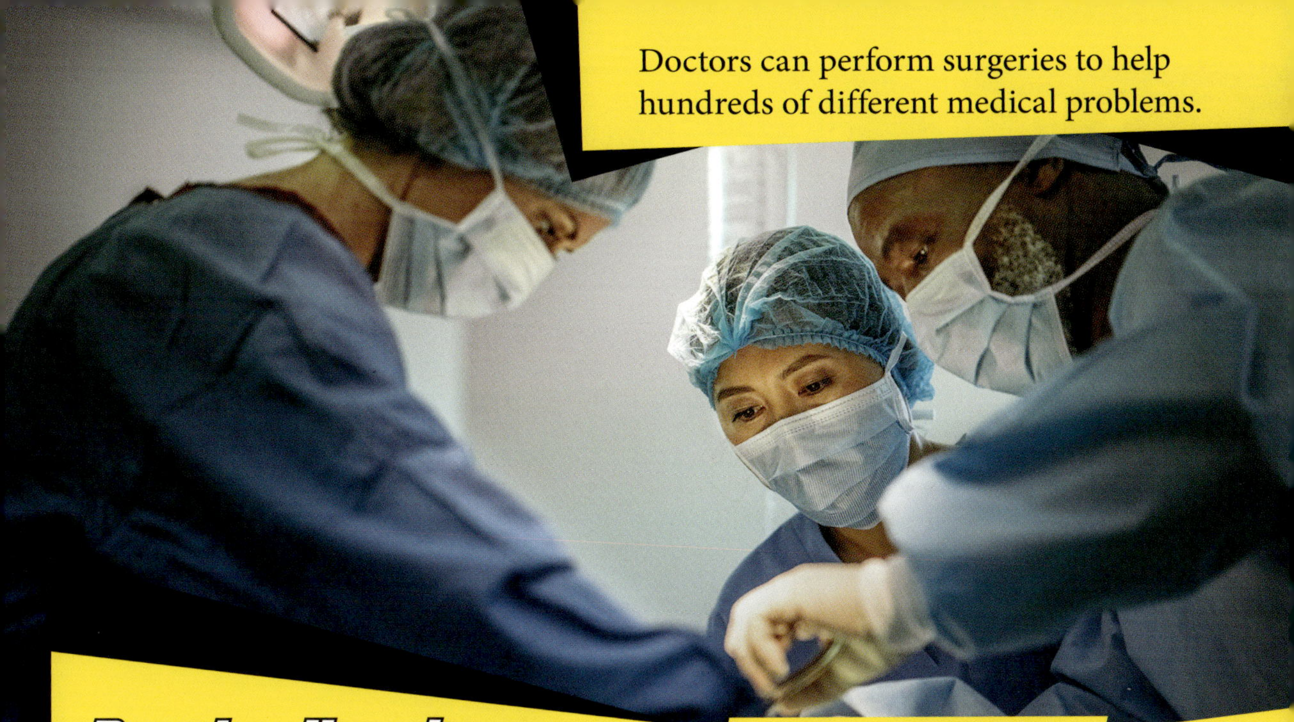

Doctors can perform surgeries to help hundreds of different medical problems.

By the Numbers

The human body contains billions of working parts. No wonder sometimes strange things happen.

60,000 miles (96,560 kilometers)

how long all the blood vessels in our body would stretch if laid out

9 to 12 pints (4.3 to 5.7 liters)

amount of blood in an average adult

5

number of organs you need to survive—brain, heart, kidneys, liver, and lungs

650

about this many muscles

206

number of bones

100 billion

about this many nerve cells in our brain

1.5 quarts (1.42 l)

the amount of urine our kidneys produce each day

3-D Printing

Imagine being able to use a printer to replace missing or damaged arms, legs, bones, or organs. This may sound more like fantasy than medicine. But 3-D printers are already being used to create medical devices. For example, scientists have printed foot braces, replacement limbs, and even dental implants. Lee Cronin, a scientist in Glasgow, Scotland, even believes that we will some day be able to 3-D print medications.

3-D printing can help the medical process in several ways. Working from a standard design, 3-D printers can create many copies of something quickly. Even better, 3-D printers make it easy to adjust the design to match a person's exact needs. The cost is also less than with a normal building process.

A 3-D printed artificial hand can help people who have lost a hand.

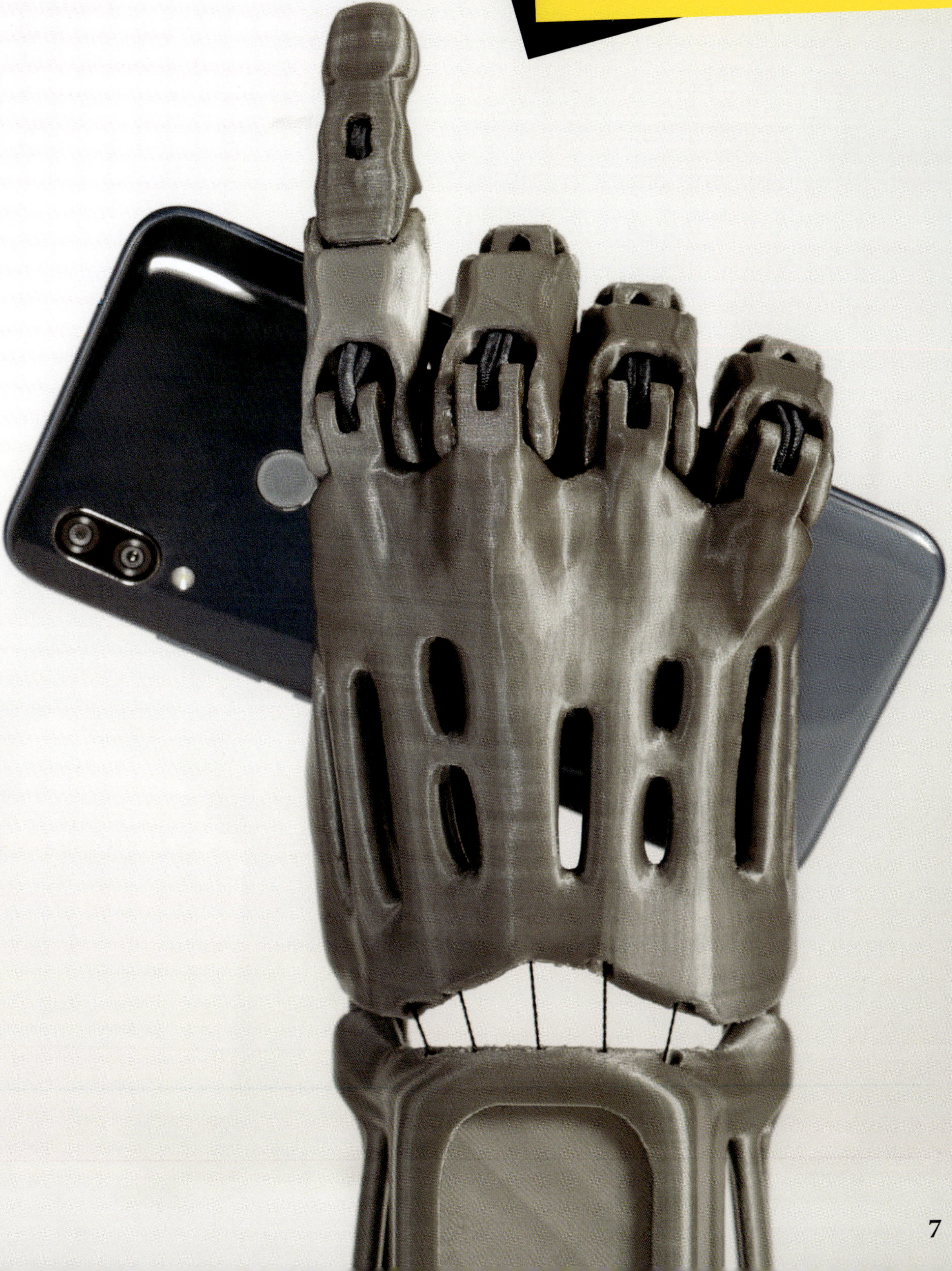

Currently, scientists can 3-D print skin and liver cells. They have printed heart valves and ear cartilage too. Many scientists believe that they will be able to print entire organs by the year 2030. This would change how organ **transplants** are done. The ability to transplant organs has saved the lives of countless people. But for many organ transplants, patients have to wait a long time for a healthy person to die and donate his or her organs.

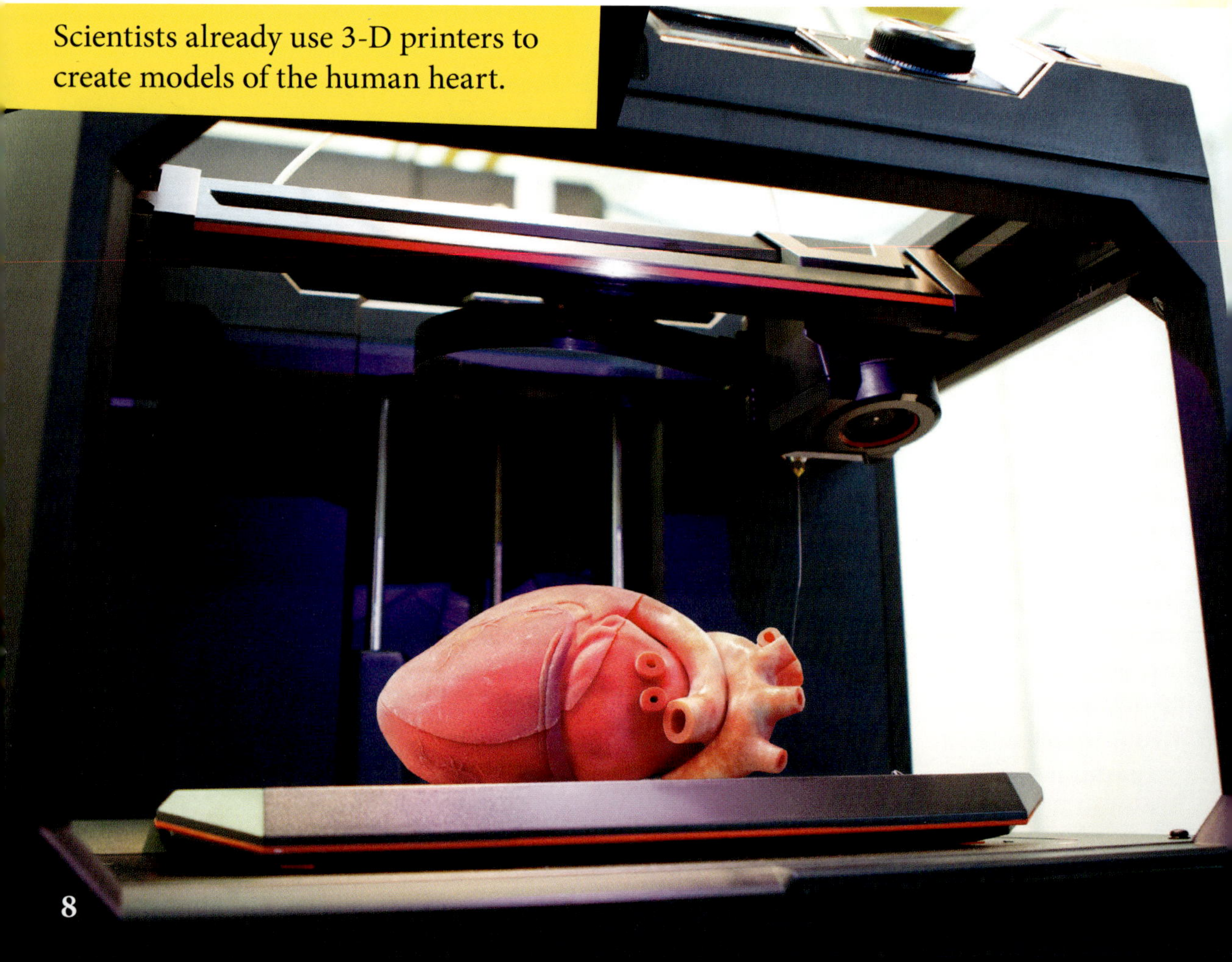

Scientists already use 3-D printers to create models of the human heart.

Fact!

Many famous movies feature people who have special abilities due to mechanical parts built into their bodies. These movies include *Justice League*, *Ghost in the Shell*, **and the** *Terminator* **movies.**

If scientists are able to 3-D print entire organs, people in need would have a much shorter wait time. They could also receive organs specifically made for their bodies instead of waiting for a donor that matches their blood type.

3-D printing technology gets better all the time. Who knows what amazing products it may produce soon? 3-D printing could one day improve or even save millions of lives!

Painful, Swollen Limbs

Elephantiasis is the name for a condition where a person's limbs swell and become hard. It's very painful, and it happens when **lymph** vessels get blocked.

More than 120 million people have some degree of this condition. It is often caused by a certain type of roundworm. It is spread by mosquitoes. Roundworm **larvae** enter the bloodstream through mosquito bites. The roundworms grow there. Over time, they damage people's lymph systems. The arms, legs, or feet may begin to swell. The skin grows thick and hard. The swollen limbs are painful.

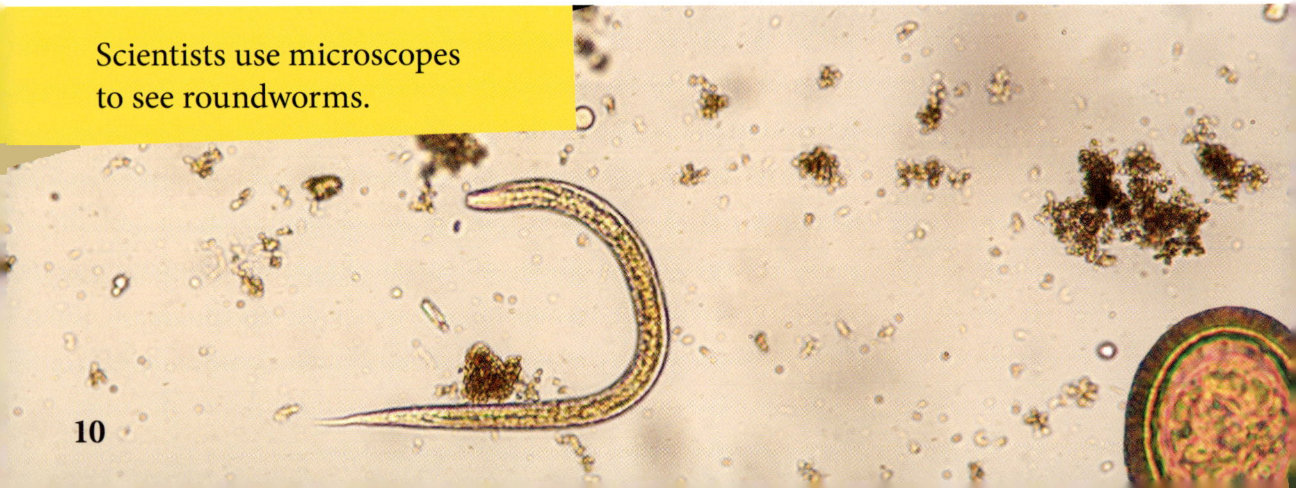

Scientists use microscopes to see roundworms.

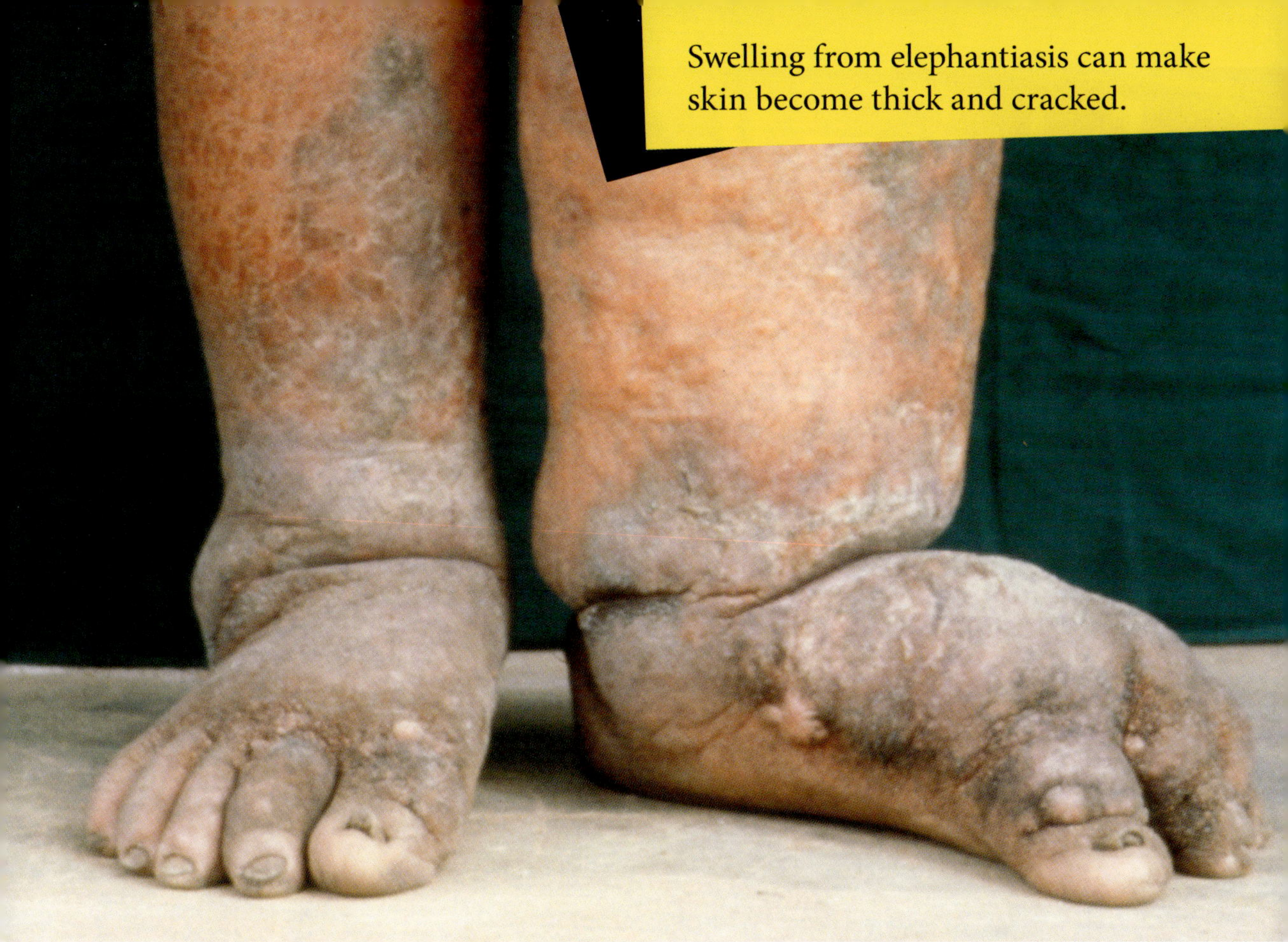

Swelling from elephantiasis can make skin become thick and cracked.

Elephantiasis happens most often in countries with warm, rainy weather. Roundworms thrive there. Millions of mosquitoes are also around to spread the disease. There is no cure, but doctors use medicine to treat the symptoms. Perhaps future discoveries can help cure people suffering with this difficult condition.

Fact!

There has not been a case of elephantiasis in the United States in 100 years.

Extreme Heights

Being tall has many advantages. You can see over crowds. You can reach high places. But when people get too tall it can cause health problems. Extreme height can run in families. If both parents are tall, the chances are greater that a child may grow to be very tall. In other cases, extreme height may be caused by having too many growth **hormones**. This can cause the person to grow both very tall and very heavy.

Just how tall can people get? Robert Wadlow of the United States was the world's tallest person ever. He stood 8 feet, 11 inches (272 centimeters) tall!

Wadlow could have dunked a basketball without even jumping. He was so tall he needed braces to support his long legs. He wore a size 37 shoe. Wadlow died at age 22.

A tailor measures Robert Wadlow to make him a suit.

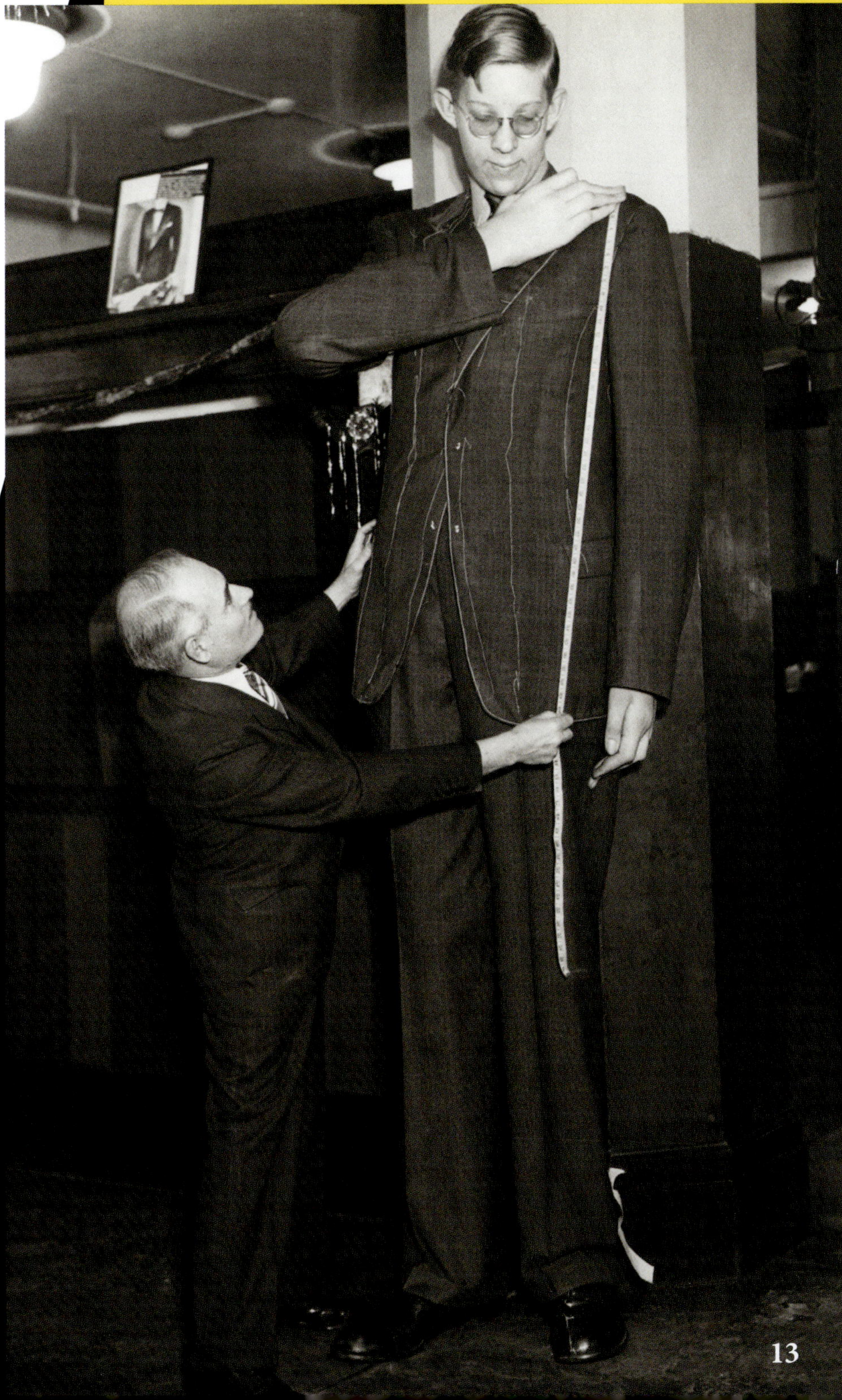

The tallest-ever woman was Zeng Jinlian of China. She stood 8 feet, 1.75 inches (248 cm) tall. She died in 1982 at the age of 17.

There are many men and several women living today who stand more than 7 feet (213 cm) tall. As of the year 2020, the tallest living person is Sultan Kösen of Turkey. He measures 8 feet, 2.8 inches (251 cm) tall. He actually had surgery to stop him from growing any taller.

Fact!

Today, the average human is about 4 inches (10 cm) taller than a person from the mid-1800s. Scientists credit this to better childhood nutrition.

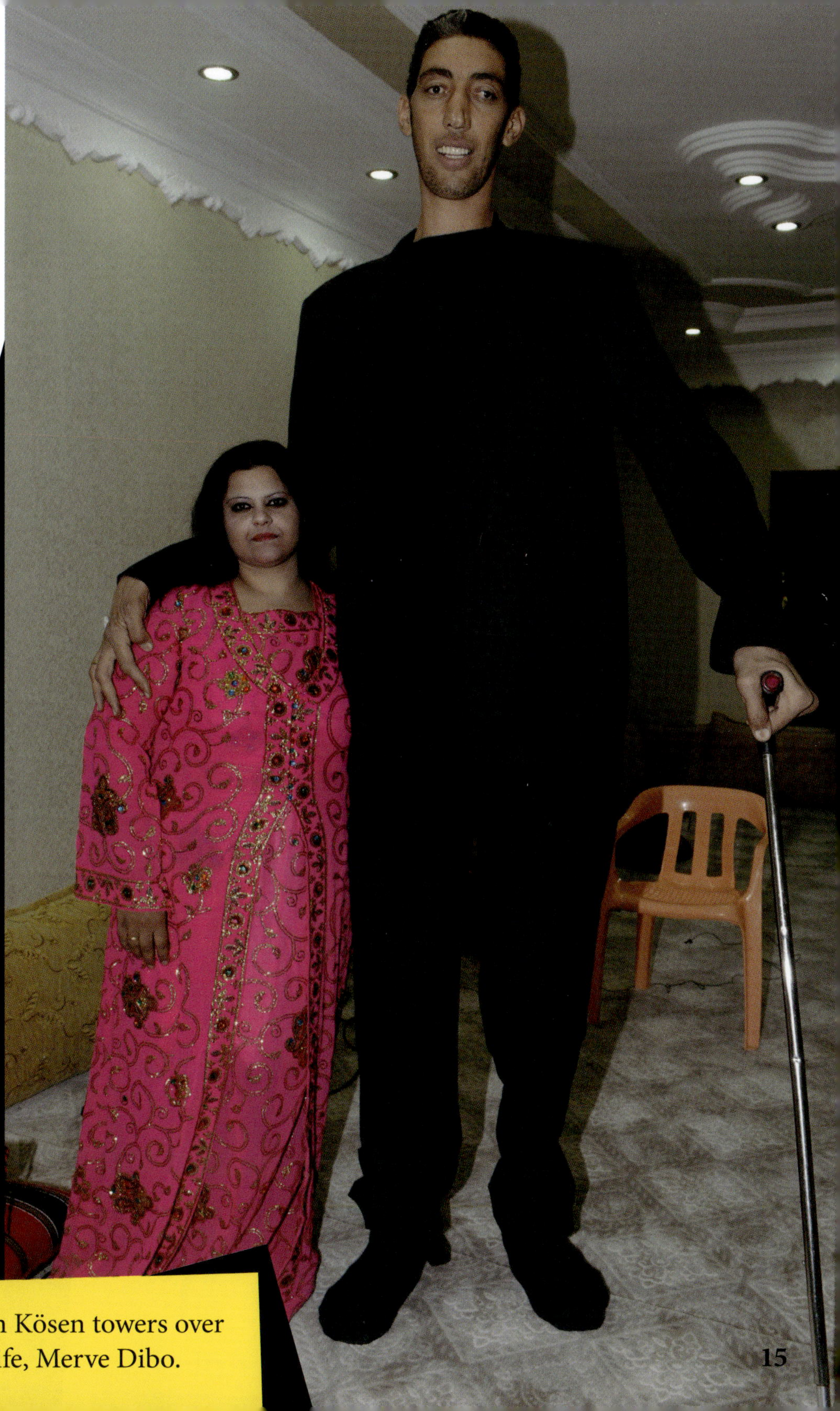

Sultan Kösen towers over his wife, Merve Dibo.

Tapeworms

Imagine having a creature 20 feet (6 m) long living inside you! In 2016, a man in China went to a clinic complaining of stomach pains. He had lost 11 pounds (5 kilograms) in just three days. Doctors studied his poop and found a tapeworm egg. The man said he often ate raw beef, which can carry tapeworms. Doctors gave him some medicine. Soon he pooped out a 20-foot (6-m) tapeworm!

A 20-foot (6-m) tapeworm is about as long as these items:

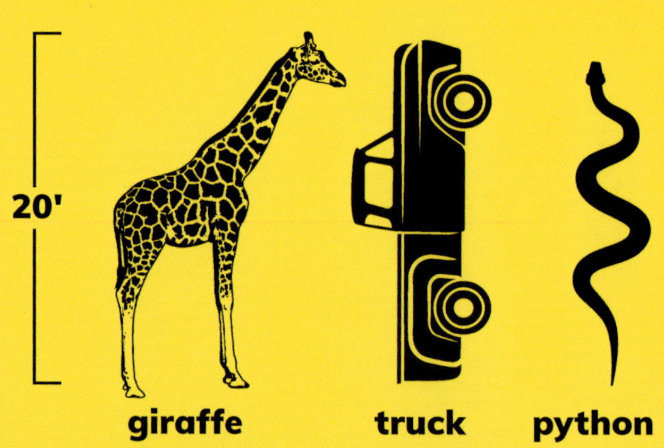

In 2019, a New York woman went to her doctor complaining of odd symptoms. She kept forgetting words and dropping things. An MRI showed a spot on her brain. Doctors feared she might have cancer. Instead, they found a baby tapeworm. Doctors had no idea how it got there. Luckily, they were able to remove the tapeworm, and the woman's symptoms improved.

Tapeworms are a type of **parasite**. These creepy creatures can get into a person's body. That's what causes the unpleasant symptoms. Humans most often catch tapeworms by eating raw beef.

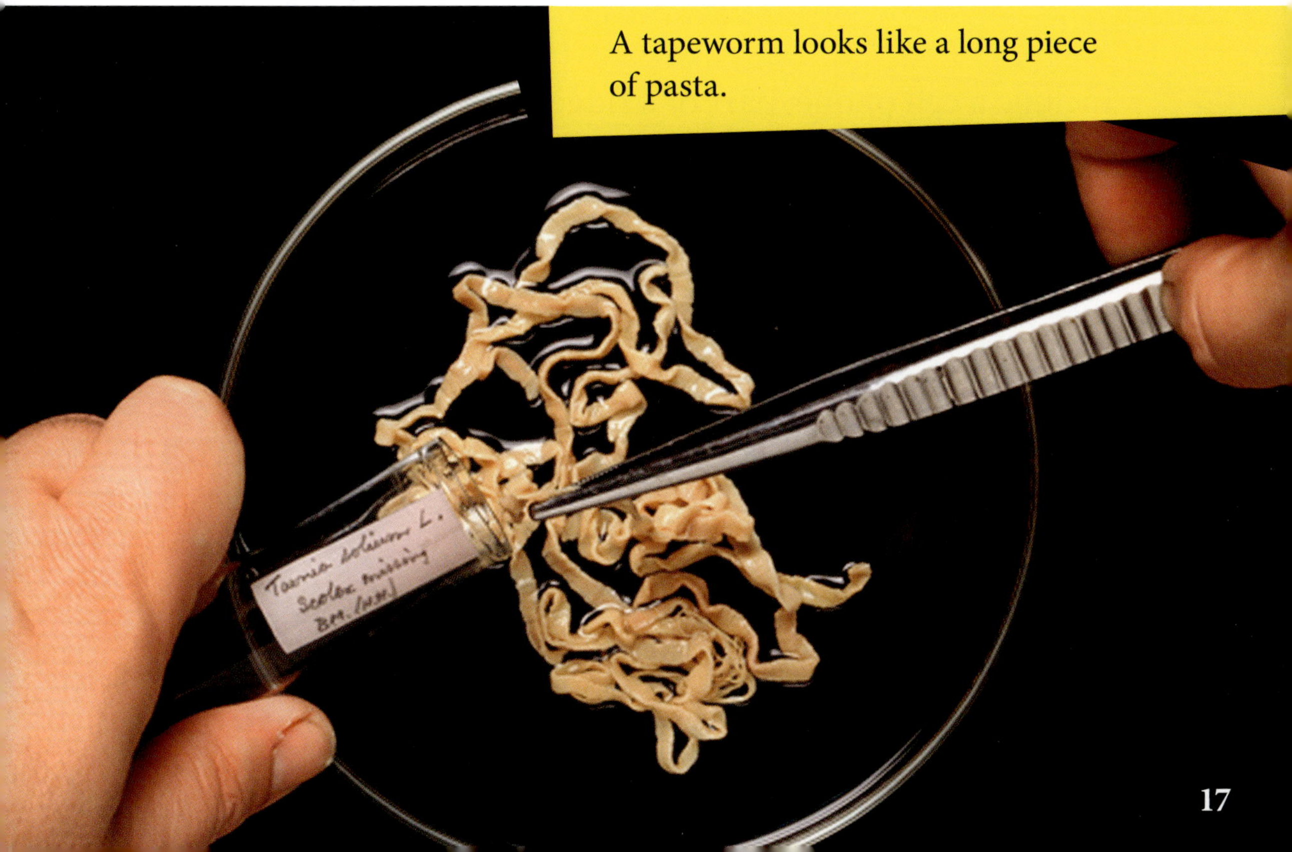

A tapeworm looks like a long piece of pasta.

They Swallowed What?

Young children sometimes swallow strange things. Coins, toys, and marbles are common offenders. Most times these objects simply pass through the child's digestive system and get pooped out. But sometimes objects can get stuck and cause serious damage.

Even adults swallow things they shouldn't. Doctors have removed some really odd items from patients of all ages. Some of the weirdest include a cell phone, part of a fidget spinner, a toothbrush, a fitness tracker, and part of a set of false teeth. Some items that go into people's stomachs pass out on their own. The process usually takes four to six days. Other items must be removed with surgery.

Fact!

Cases of children swallowing strange objects in the United States nearly doubled between 1995 and 2015. More than 40,000 cases were reported in 2015.

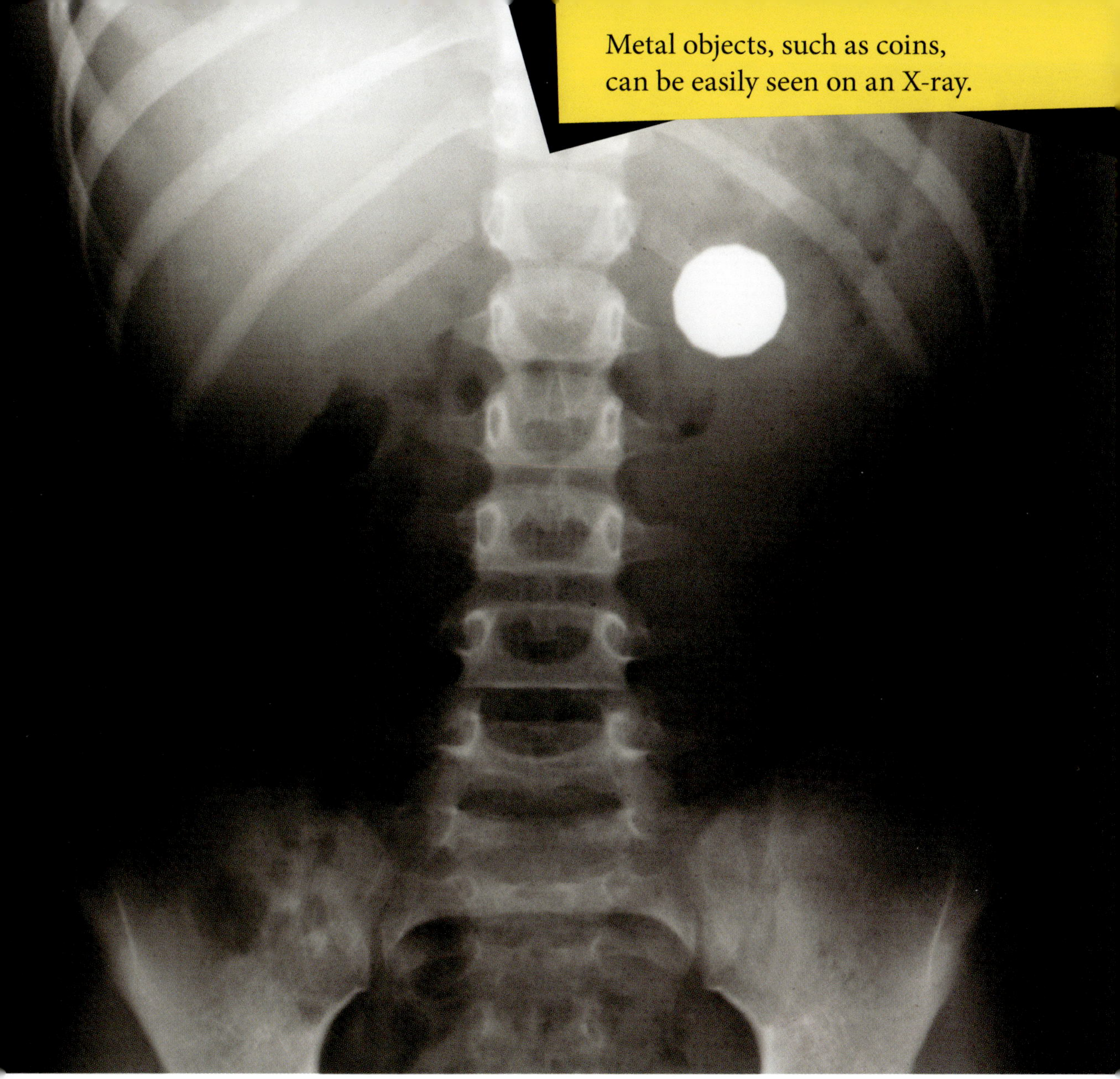

Metal objects, such as coins, can be easily seen on an X-ray.

In some cases, doctors can easily remove an item from the patient's throat. Removing objects from a person's throat is a lot like fishing. Doctors use snares, nets, and other tools. Most patients recover completely.

Blood-Sucking Leeches

You're sick. What would you think if the doctor placed a slimy leech on your body to suck your blood?

Leeches are a type of worm. They live in lakes, ponds, and rivers. They attach to other creatures and feed on their blood. Leeches have suckers at each end of their body. That is how they attach to a **host**. Then they use their sharp teeth to bite the host and suck its blood. When they finish eating, they simply let go and fall off.

Doctors have used leeches to treat disease for thousands of years. Early doctors thought many diseases were the result of too much blood or "bad blood" in the body. They used leeches to draw blood from people. Doctors used leeches to treat everything from headaches to toothaches to serious diseases.

In the United States, doctors used leeches throughout the 1700s and 1800s. Leeches were so popular that people in Europe grew them on farms and sold them. Sometimes draining blood did reduce fever. But it also weakened the patient. Often it did more harm than good. By the mid-1900s, few doctors used them anymore. They found modern medicines worked better.

Hundreds of years ago, doctors had many ways to let out "bad blood." Sometimes they would make a small cut to release blood.

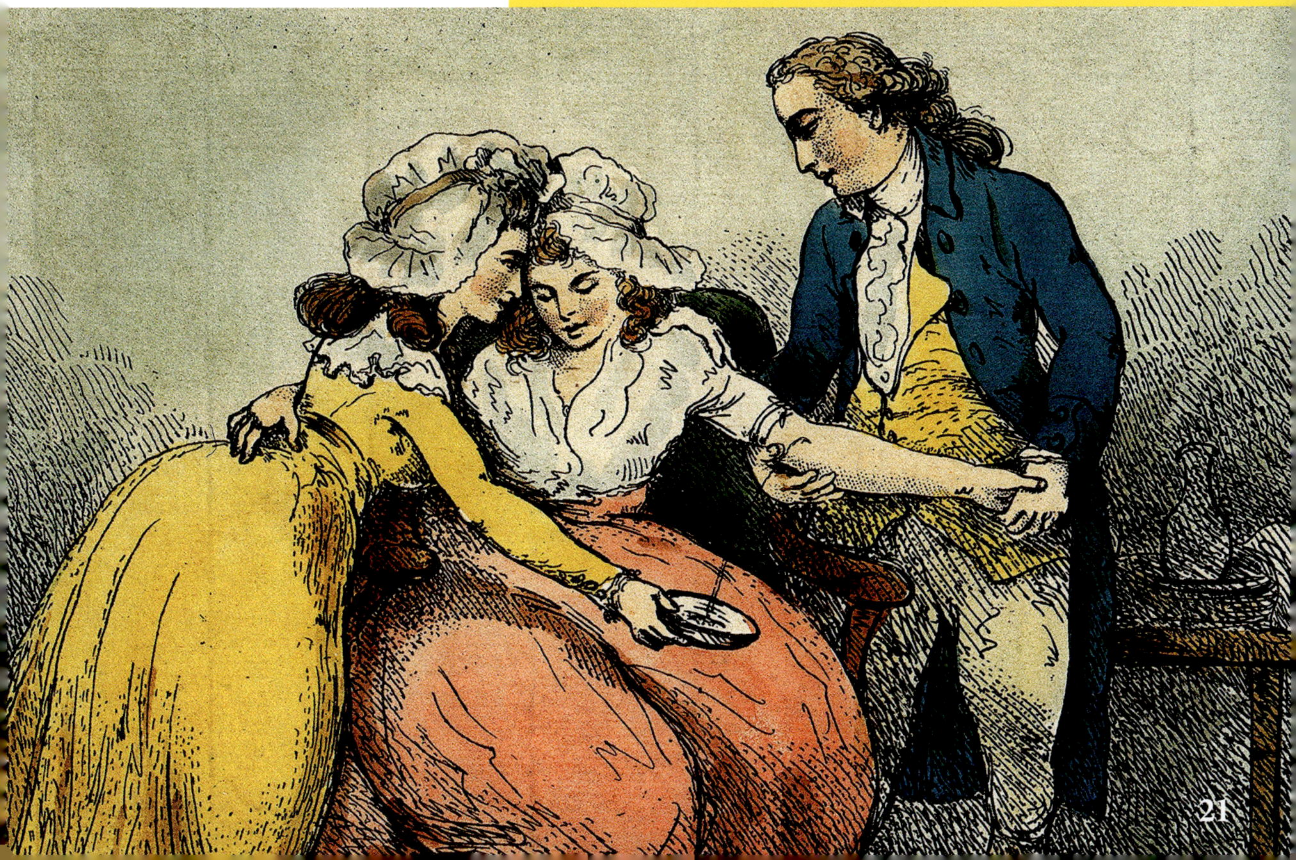

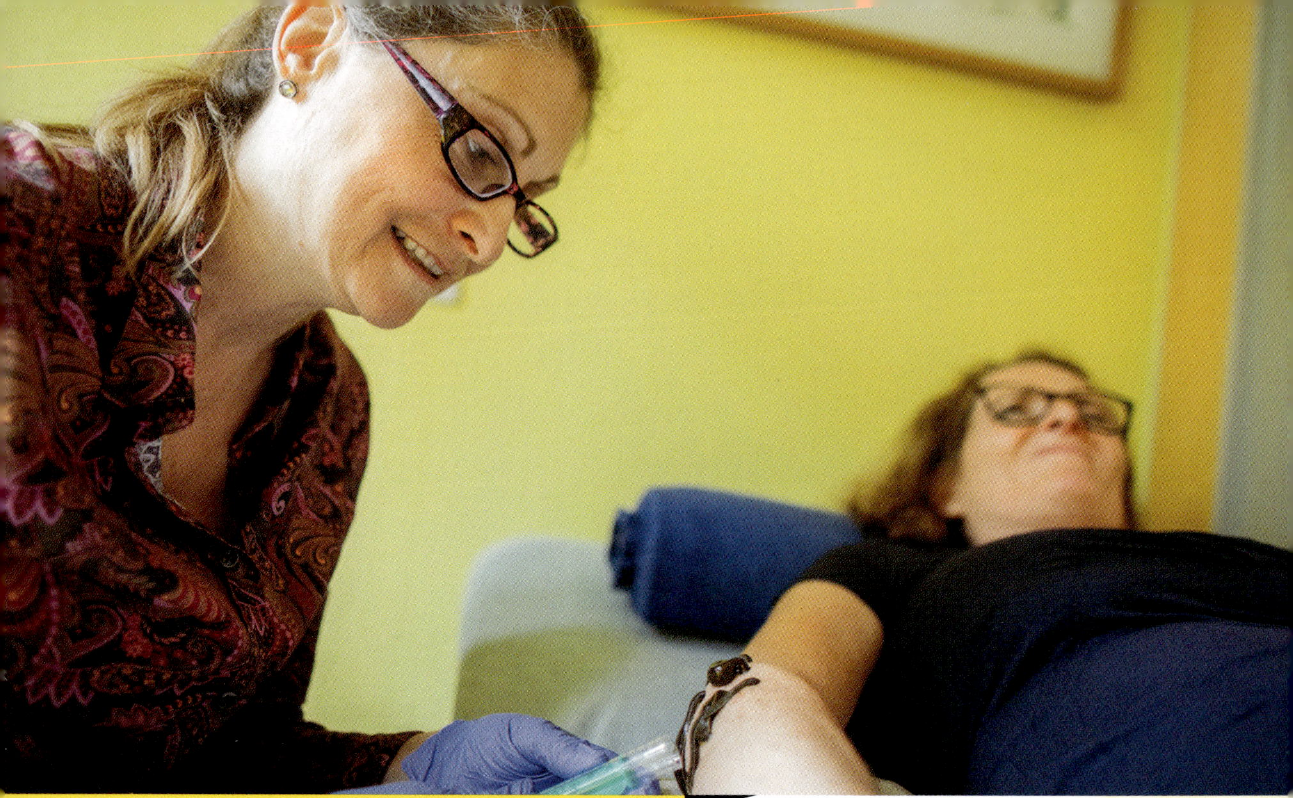

A German doctor places leeches on her patient.

Today, leeches are making a comeback. Doctors use them to treat certain problems. Leeches can help when doctors reattach a limb. After the surgery, blood flows to the reattached limb through blood vessels called arteries. But sometimes the vessels that carry blood away are not yet working. This causes the limb to swell and turn blue. Leeches can remove the excess blood. This gives the body time to get its own vessels working again.

Fact!

Some leeches are less than 1 inch (2.5 cm) long. Others can grow to nearly 1.5 feet (0.3 m) in length. Smaller leeches are the ones used for medical treatments.

Leeches are also used to heal infected wounds. They eat the dead tissue so that wounds can heal. Maybe you can't imagine letting a doctor put one on your body. But leeches really can help save lives.

In India, leeches are used to treat an itchy foot condition called chilblains.

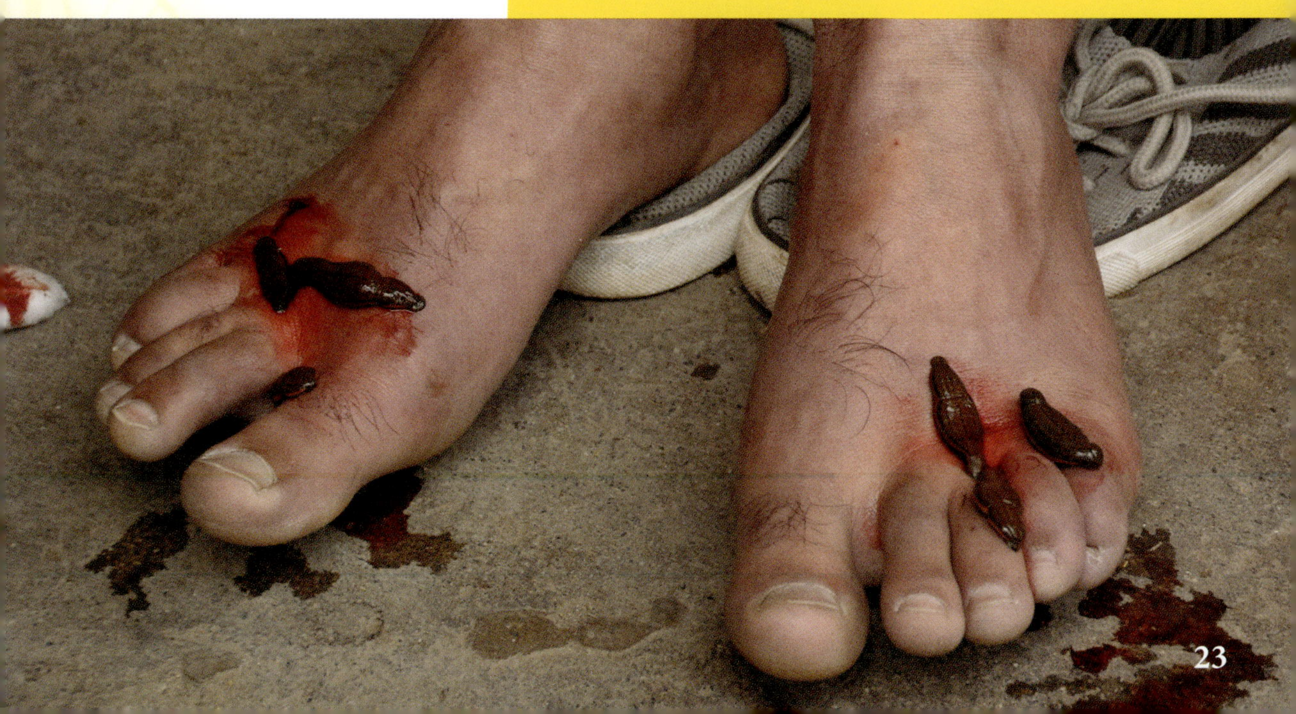

Crabs in Labs

Horseshoe crabs have a tank-like body, a long, spiny tail, and multiple sets of eyes. They will probably never make it onto a list of cute creatures. Yet their blood can save human lives. The crabs' blood carries special cells. When these cells come in contact with substances called endotoxins, they make the crab's blood clot.

Why does that matter to people? Endotoxins can cause humans to have severe fevers or even organ failure. Sometimes these endotoxins can get into drugs or needles. The crab's blood can be used to test if endotoxins are present in certain drugs and medical equipment. This can save people's lives.

Fact!

How valuable is horseshoe crab blood? One quart (0.9 l) is worth more than $15,000.

Horseshoe crabs may not need to give their blood for much longer. Scientists have created a man-made substitute that does the same thing as horseshoe crab blood. This drug has been around for more than 15 years. It is slowly gaining popularity. Over time, it may replace the need for horseshoe crab blood. Then the crabs will no longer have to be blood donors.

Researchers draw blood from horseshoe crabs in a lab.

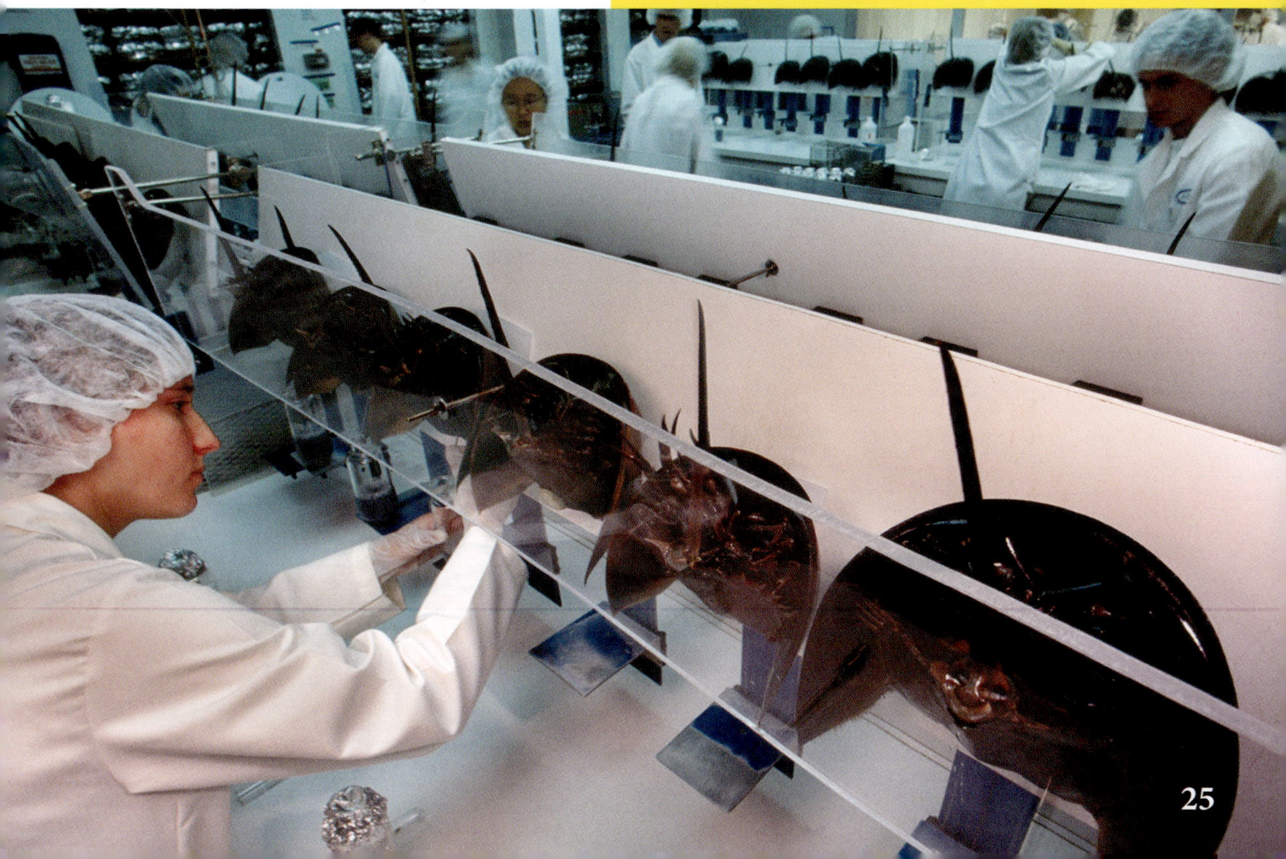

Cancer-Sniffing Beagles

You probably know that dogs have sensitive noses. Their sense of smell is 10,000 times better than that of humans. Some dogs have been trained to sniff out illegal drugs. Others sniff for bombs in airports. A recent study shows that specially trained beagles may be able to smell lung cancer!

Researchers trained three dogs for several weeks. Then they had the dogs sniff blood samples. Some of the samples came from healthy people. Others came from people with lung cancer. The dogs were trained to sit if they smelled cancer in a sample. The dogs were accurate more than 95 percent of the time.

Fact!

Non-small cell lung cancer is the second most common type of cancer in the United States. It also causes more deaths than any other cancer.

Now these researchers are training the dogs to sniff out other types of cancer as well. Finding cancer early means better treatment. Over time, trained dogs might be able to save thousands of lives!

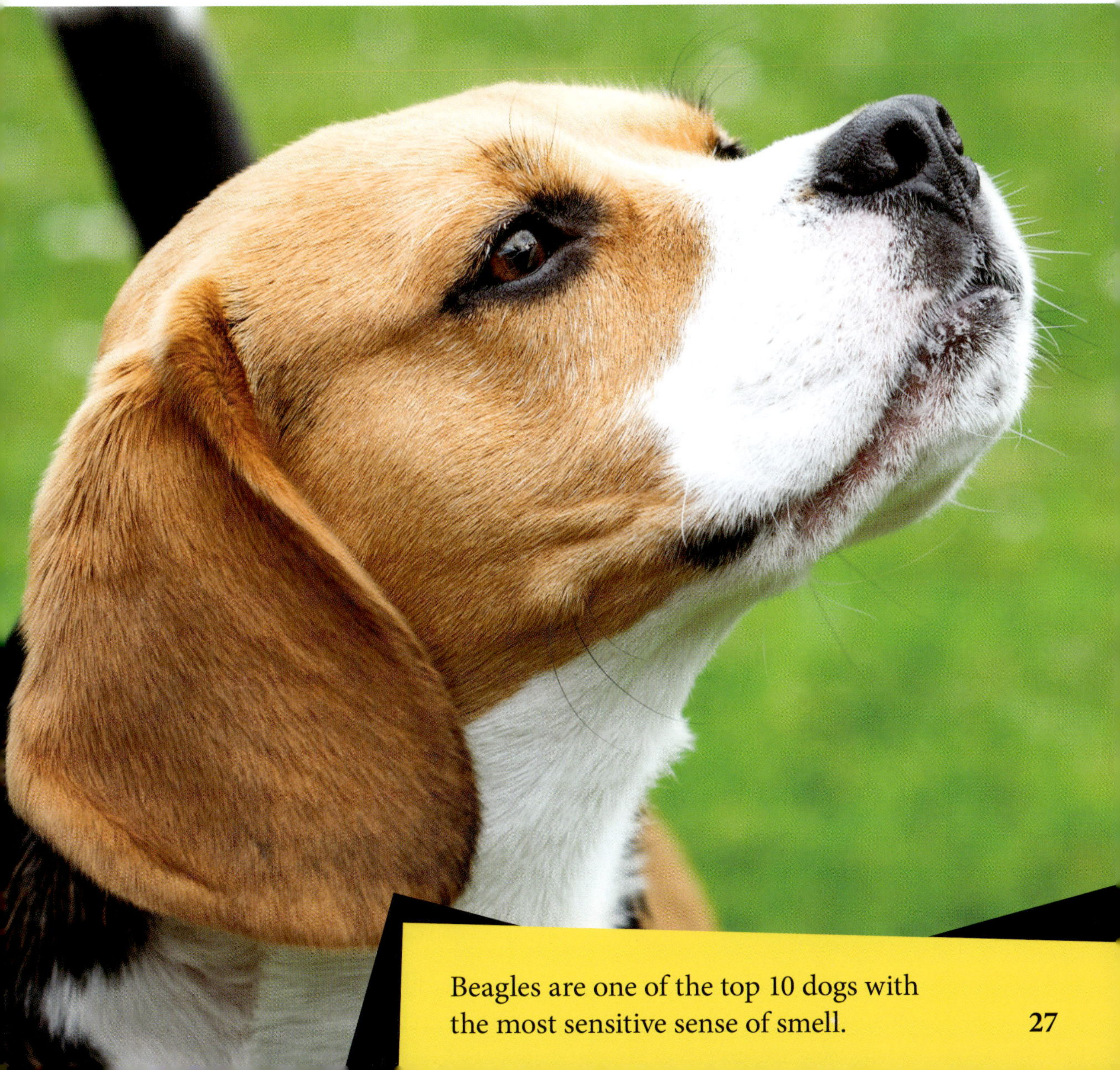

Beagles are one of the top 10 dogs with the most sensitive sense of smell.

On Pins and Needles

Don't like needles? You're not alone. The fear of needles ranks among the top **phobias** that people have. So why do so many people use **acupuncture** as a treatment for pain and disease? Acupuncture involves sticking thin needles into the skin in specific places.

This treatment has many uses. Some people use it to reduce the pain from headaches or backaches. Some use it to ease dental pain. Some use it to treat joint pain or allergies. Others use it to reduce cancer pain. Many people report feeling relief after just one or two treatments.

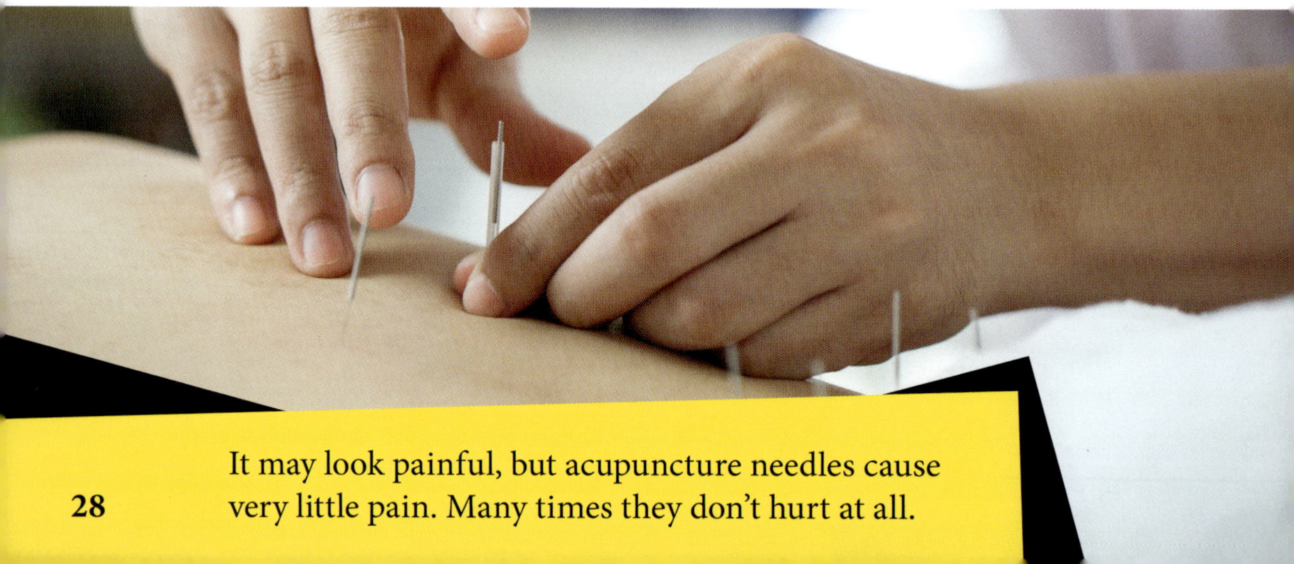

It may look painful, but acupuncture needles cause very little pain. Many times they don't hurt at all.

Acupuncture has been popular in China for thousands of years. Now it's becoming popular worldwide. Millions of Americans get acupuncture every year.

Most Common Phobias

Fear of needles ranks high among people's phobias. Here are the top 10 phobias, according to a ranking by WorldAtlas. Do you fear any of these?

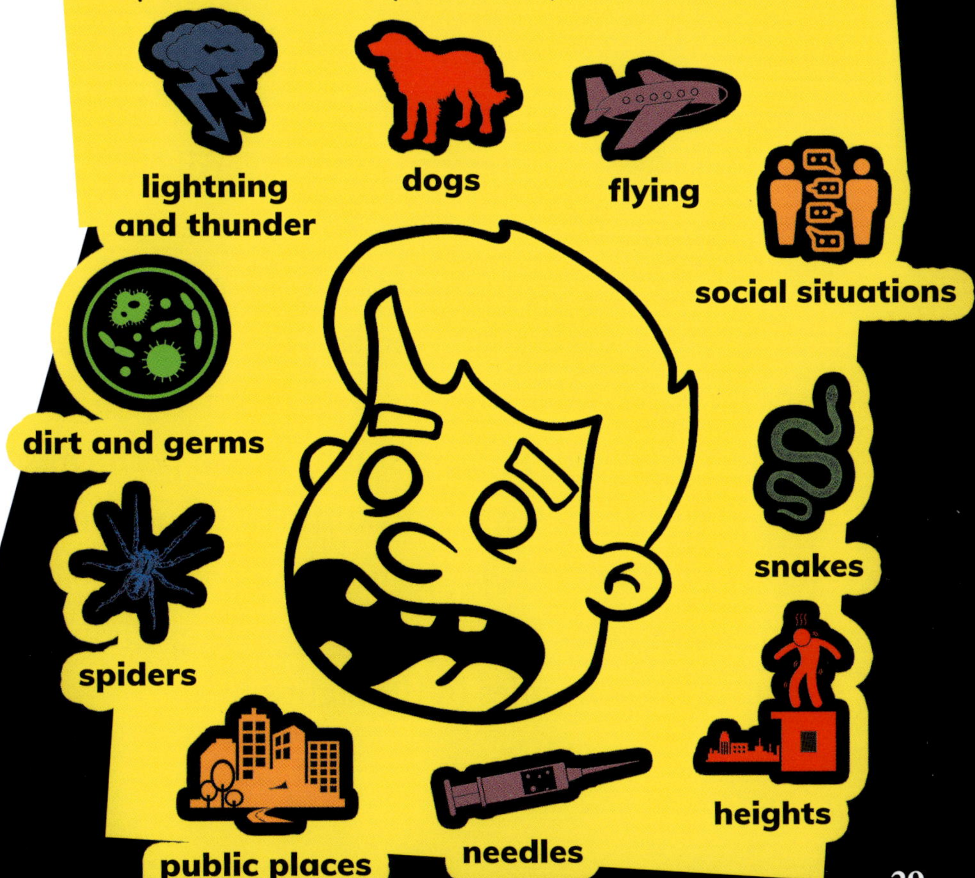
lightning and thunder
dogs
flying
social situations
dirt and germs
snakes
spiders
heights
public places
needles

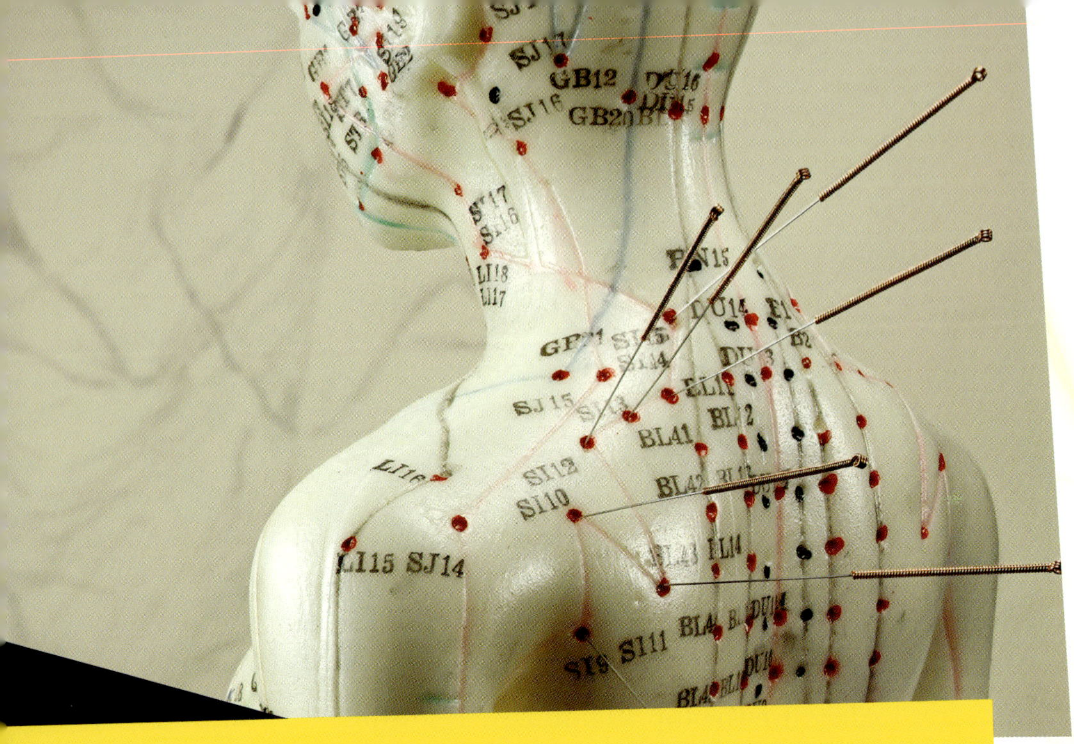

Maps of the human body show acupuncturists where to put the needles for different treatments.

How does acupuncture work? Needles are placed at certain places on the body to increase energy flow. To begin, a specially trained person asks about the patient's health history and symptoms. Then the specialist checks the shape, color, and coating of the patient's tongue. This person may also perform some other physical tests. The examination and the tests help determine where the needles should be placed. Patients lay on a treatment table. The specialist gently places needles in the right spots.

Does acupuncture hurt? Most patients say no. Some say it feels a little like a mosquito bite. Others report a feeling of heaviness or a slight, brief ache. Some feel tingly. Many people feel warm. Still others feel nothing at all. Whatever you feel at the moment, the goal is that the treatment will leave you feeling better afterward.

Some people get acupuncture in their face.

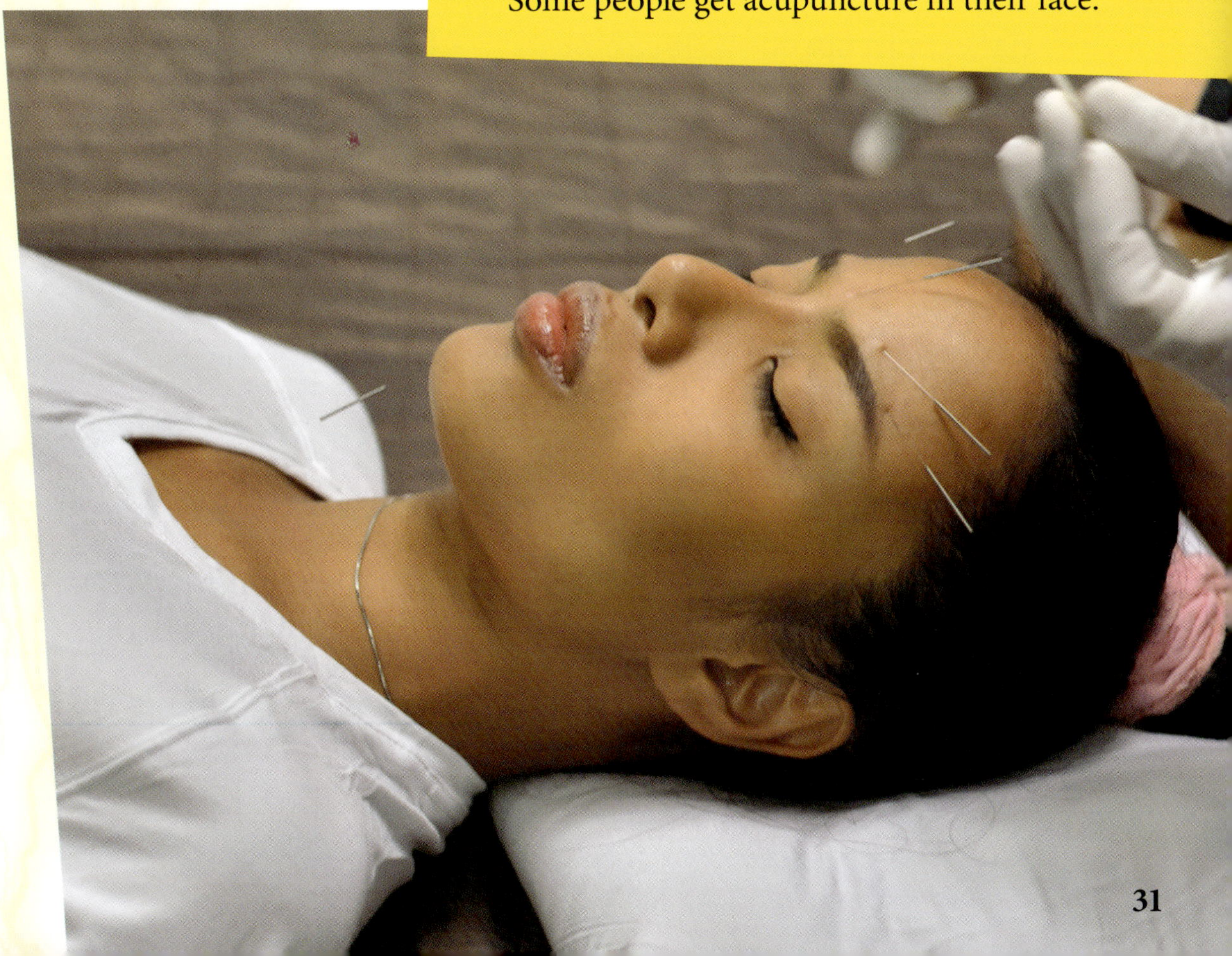

Healing Venom

Most snakes are harmless, but some carry deadly venom. A single bite from a cobra, black mamba, or rattlesnake can seriously harm or kill a person. However, the venom from certain kinds of creatures, including snakes, can also heal. It can be used to treat diseases or ease pain.

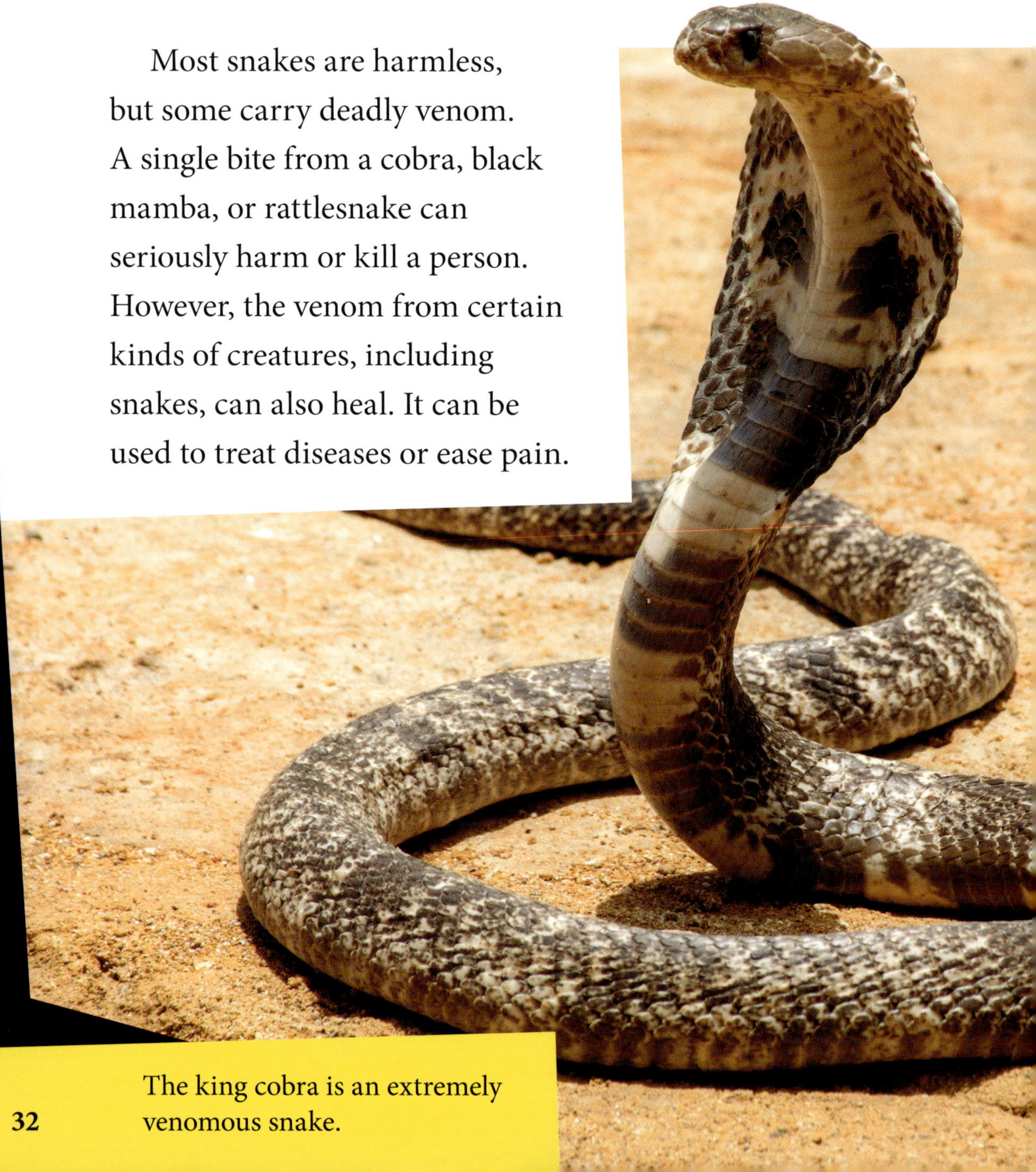

The king cobra is an extremely venomous snake.

The same things that make snake venom deadly can also turn it into a medicine. Snake venom attacks cells and tissue. It can cause **paralysis**, internal bleeding, and stop the heart. But snake venom can also be used to treat heart disease.

One heart disease drug is based on the venom of pit vipers. Mixed with other chemicals, it can treat high blood pressure. Drugs based on rattlesnake venom can help prevent the blood clots that cause heart attacks and strokes. A drug based on the venom of the deadly black mamba is being tested as a pain killer.

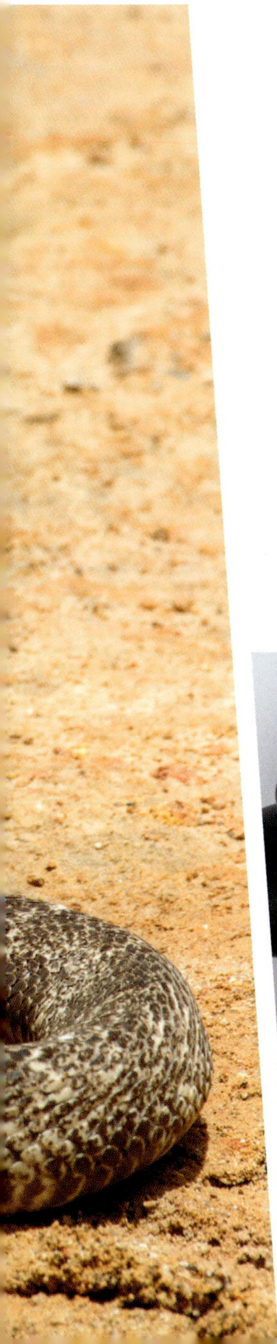

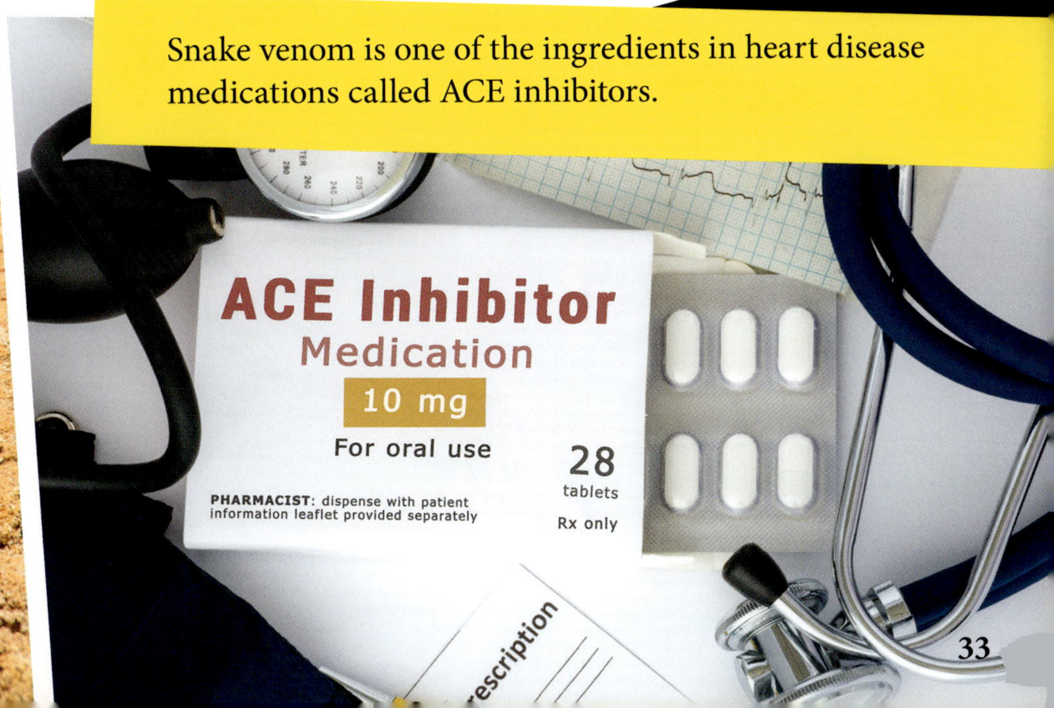

Snake venom is one of the ingredients in heart disease medications called ACE inhibitors.

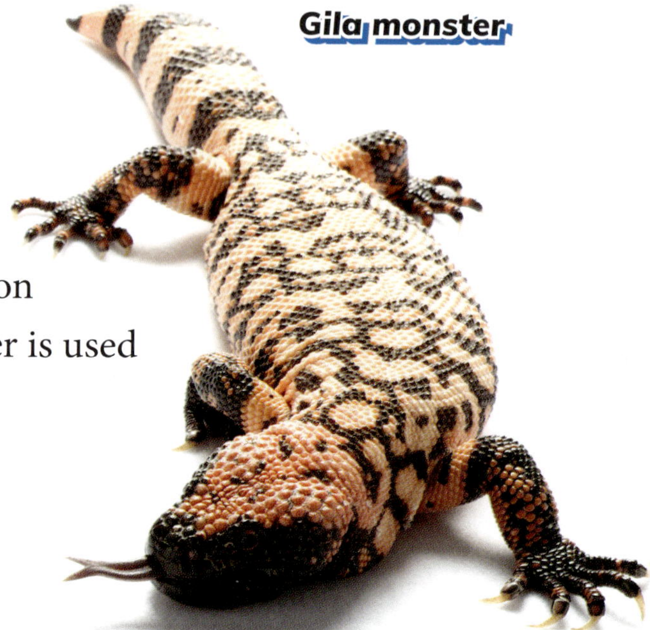

Gila monster

Other creatures also make poisons with healing properties. Medicine based on the **toxin** of the Gila monster is used to treat **diabetes**.

The U.S. Food and Drug Administration (FDA) has already approved six drugs based on animal venom. Many more are being developed. Researchers are studying how scorpion venom can help surgeons target cancerous brain cells more effectively. "Painting" these cells would let surgeons target them better. Surgeons could take out all of the cancer cells without removing healthy brain cells.

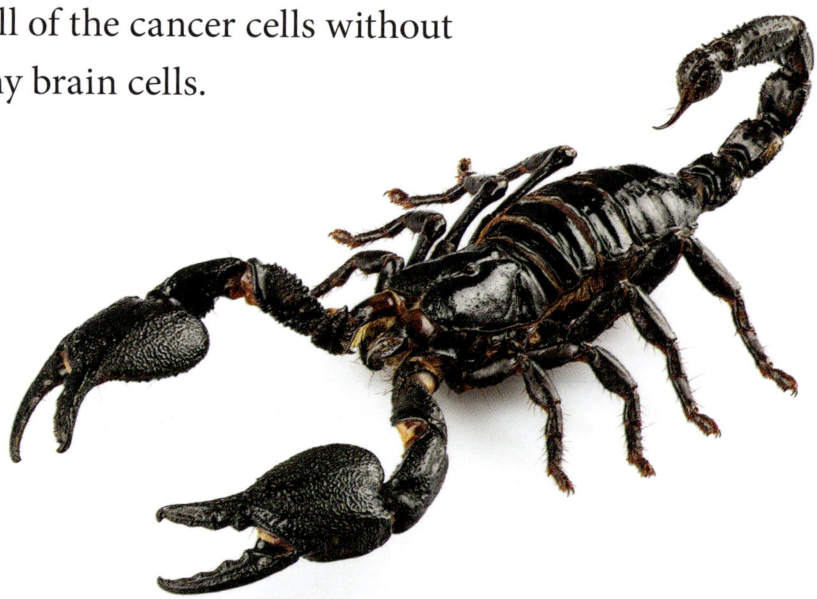

scorpion

Lots of Venom!

According to scientists, more than 150,000 animals can directly poison other creatures. Some do it as a way to get food. Others do it for defense. The 10 most venomous creatures on Earth are:

1. Scorpions
2. Chilean Recluse Spider
3. Black Widow Spider
4. Black Mamba Snake
5. Blue-ringed Octopus
6. Golden Poison Frog
7. Dubois' Sea Snake
8. Stonefish
9. Inland Taipan Snake
10. Sea Wasp

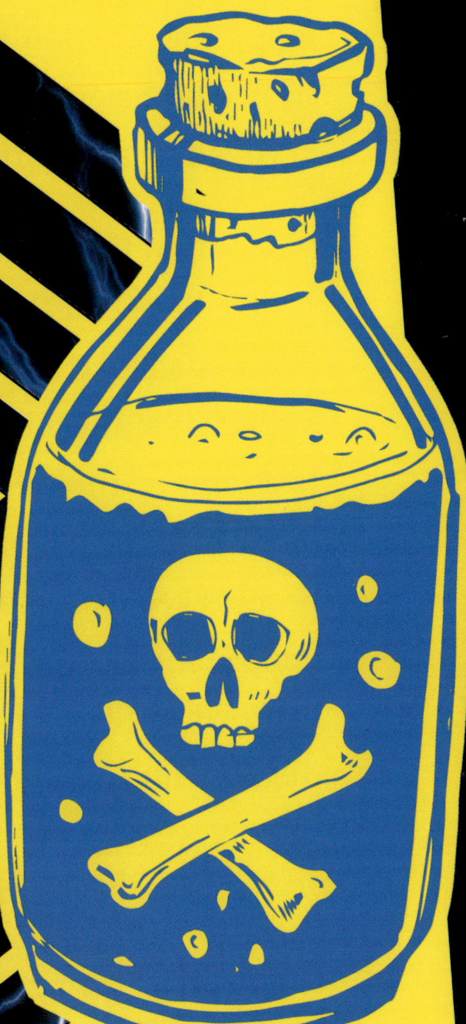

Bodies on Ice

The idea of bringing people back from the dead has been around for a long time. But could it really be done someday? Scientists in the field of **cryogenics** are working on it!

Around the world, hundreds of people have had their bodies frozen. Scientists replace the water in cells with a special liquid. Then the body is chilled to a temperature of about -220 degrees Fahrenheit (-140 degrees Celsius). This process keeps the cells from dying. People hope that someday they can be unfrozen and cured of whatever they died from.

Fact!

One of the most famous people to be cryogenically frozen is Hall of Fame baseball legend Ted Williams.

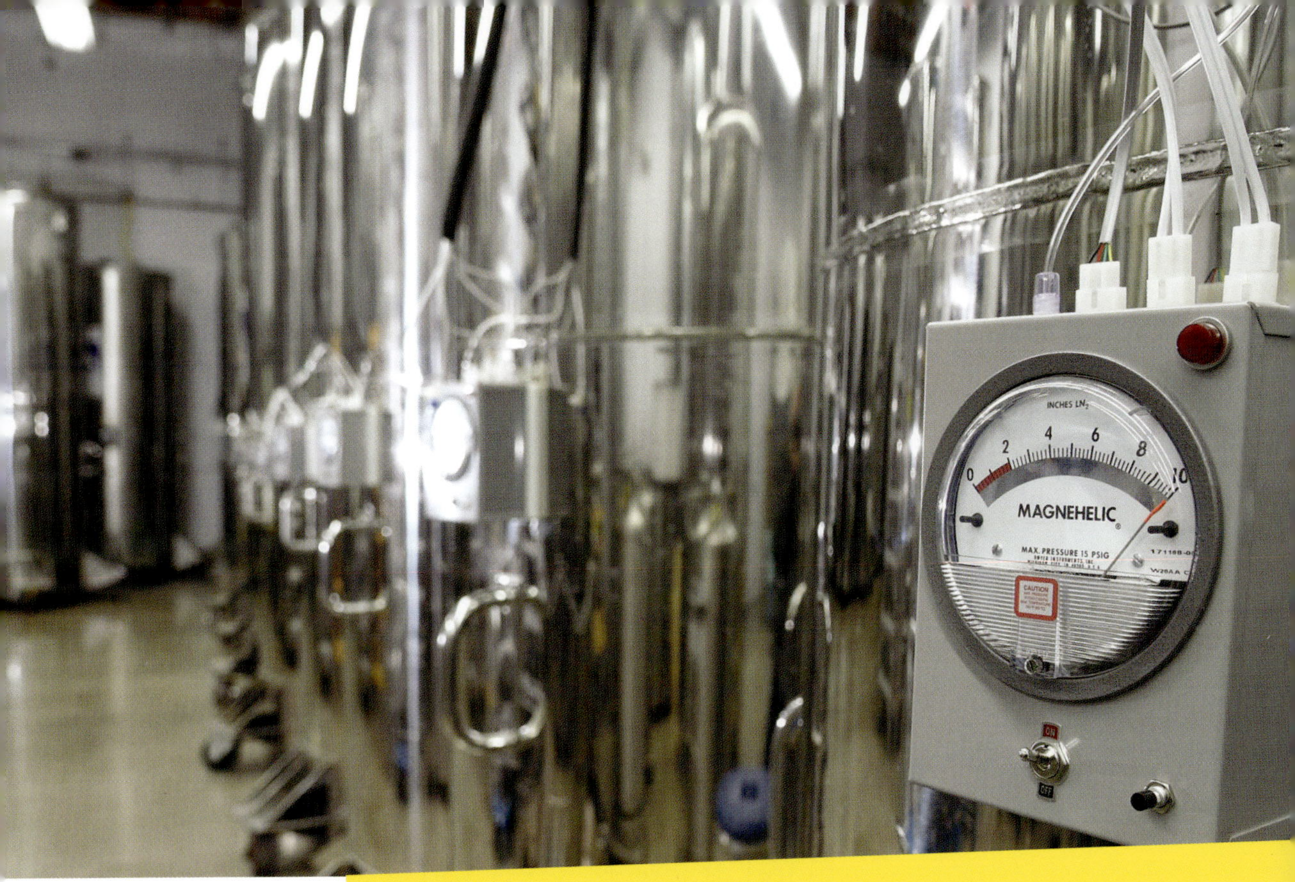

Cryogenically frozen bodies are kept in special containers.

As of now, no one knows for sure if this will work. Scientists have already thawed small amounts of tissue. The next step would be to freeze and thaw entire organs. At some point, scientists may be able to thaw entire human bodies and bring them back to life.

Laughing Your Way to Health

Have you heard the saying, "Laughter is the best medicine?" Laughter relaxes our muscles and makes us feel good. But can it really improve our health? Science proves that laughter lessens stress-causing hormones in our blood. It lowers our blood pressure. It can help fight sadness. It can ease pain too.

Dr. Madan Kataria of India created an exercise program called Laughter Yoga in the 1990s. Combining yoga and humor was a hit! It started with just a handful of people meeting in a park in Mumbai, India. Soon, many others joined the fun. Now laughter yoga has spread worldwide. Kataria's book, *Laugh for No Reason*, is available in seven languages.

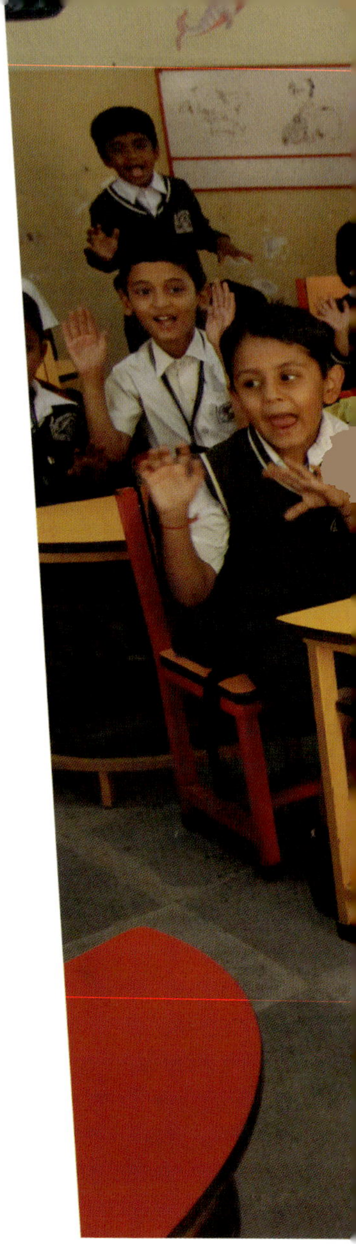

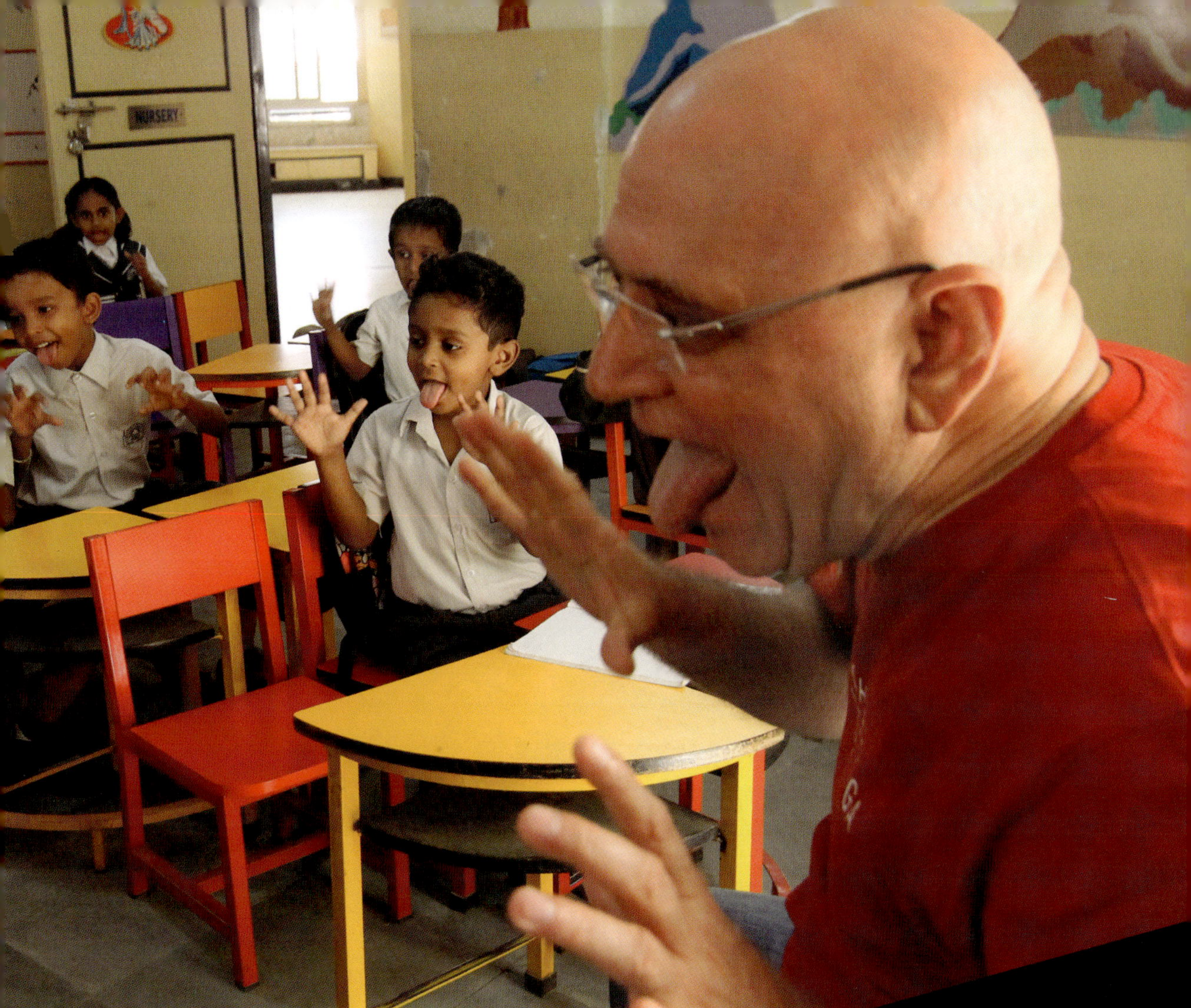

Dr. Kataria speaks to a classroom of children in India about how laughing helps to keep people healthy.

Are you looking for a simple way to feel better in both your body and your mind? Try laughter yoga exercises.

Full-Face Transplant

It started as a normal day. Then came a moment that changed Charla Nash's life forever. In February 2009, Nash was helping her friend Sandy Herold, with Herold's 200-pound (91-kg) pet chimpanzee, Travis. Suddenly, Travis went wild. He ripped off Nash's hands, nose, lips, and eyelids before being stopped by police. The attack left Nash badly injured and blind.

Surgeons tried to transplant new hands and a new face onto Nash. The surgery took 20 hours. Nash became one of only a handful of people to have ever had a successful full-face transplant. Unfortunately, the hand transplant failed.

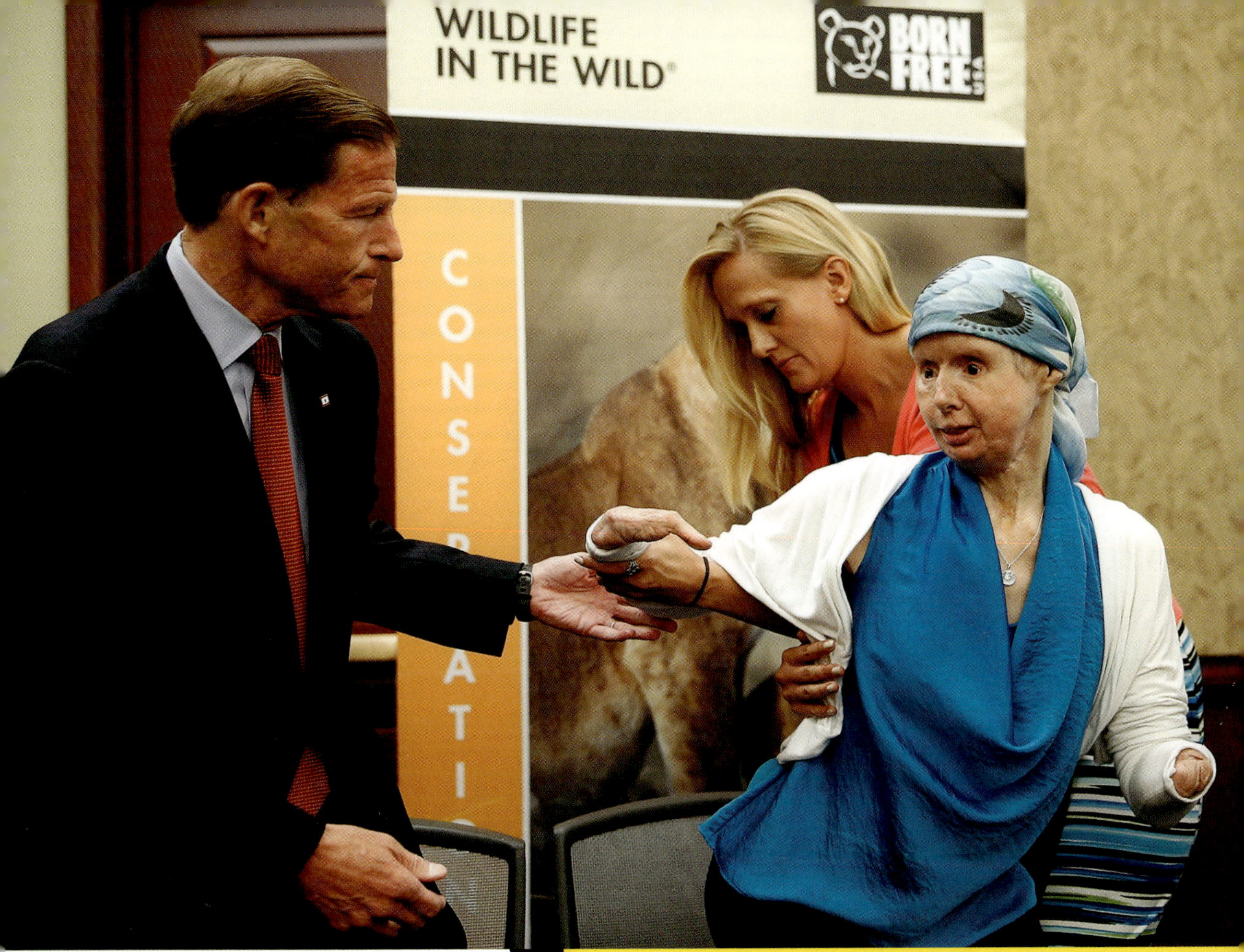

Charla Nash now helps promote laws about keeping wild animals in the wild.

Over time, Nash made great progress. In 2016, she suffered a setback. Her body started to reject her transplanted face. Once doctors changed her medications, things returned to normal. Today, Nash lives on her own in an apartment. Her life will never be the same as before the attack. Still, she is thankful to be alive.

From Dreams to Reality

Most people will face a medical challenge at some point in their lives. It could be a disease or illness. It might be an injury. Whatever happens, it's good to know that doctors and scientists are always coming up with new treatments. They are constantly working to help people with their medical issues, no matter how common or rare. By combining science and creativity, there's no limit to what hardworking health care providers may be able to treat.

Fifty years ago, doctors hardly imagined some of today's treatments. Replacing someone's face was unheard of. Printing 3-D limbs seemed like an impossible dream. Those dreams have become reality. What medical treatments might become real in another 50 years? Only time will tell!

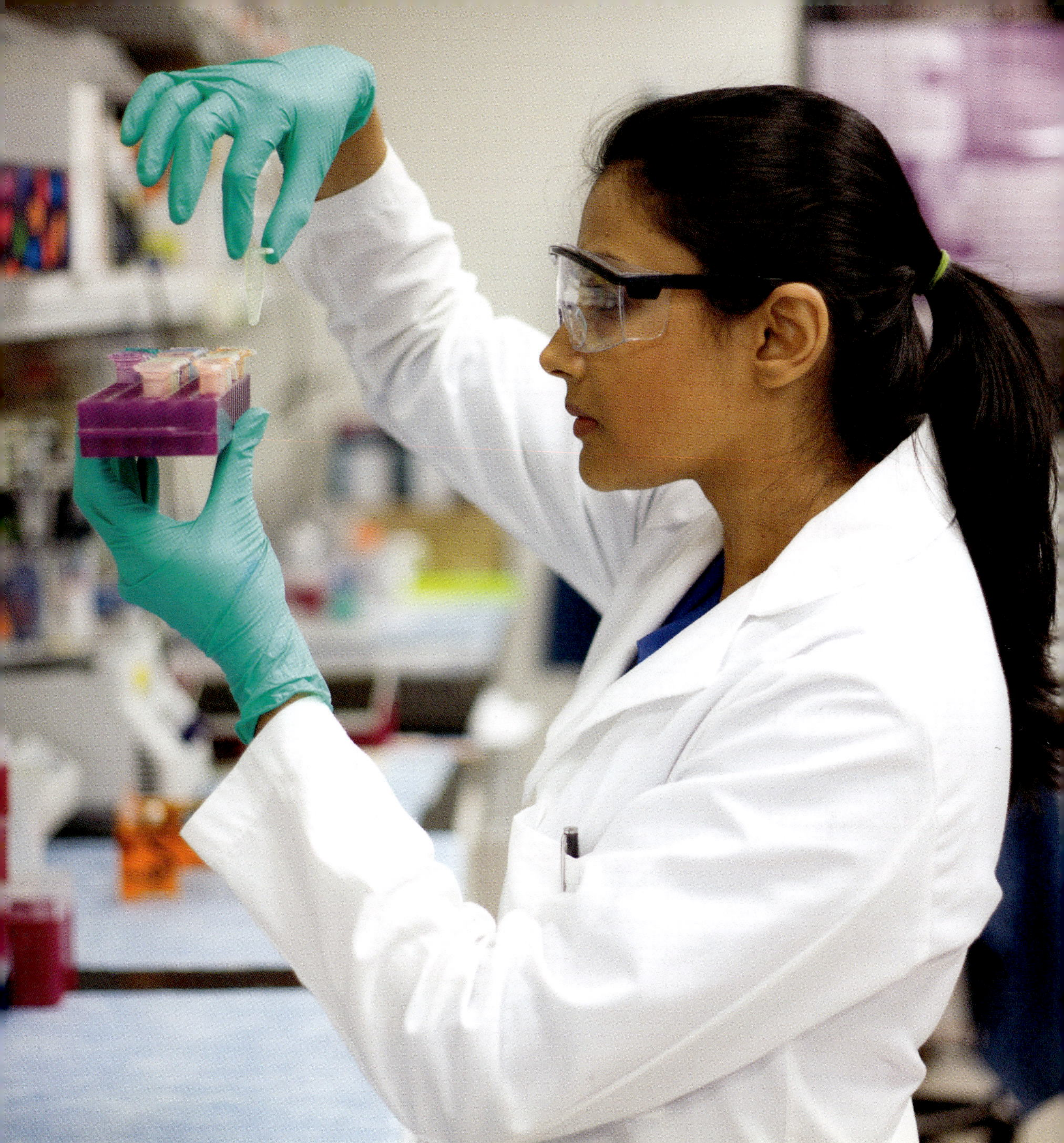

Scientists are always studying new medicines and treatments for diseases.

BUT WAIT... THERE'S MORE

GENE THERAPY

Genes are the instructions for our cells. Gene therapy is a type of medical treatment. It involves replacing harmful genes in cells with normal genes. This means doctors can treat a disease or disorder without using surgery or drugs. Gene therapy can help a patient's system fight cancer. It also can be used to treat certain types of vision problems that lead to blindness.

GIGANTIC TUMOR

Surgeons don't just remove weird things that people have swallowed. They also cut out dangerous growths called tumors that threaten people's lives. In 1991, doctors removed a tumor weighing 300 pounds (136 kg) from a woman. The surgery took six hours.

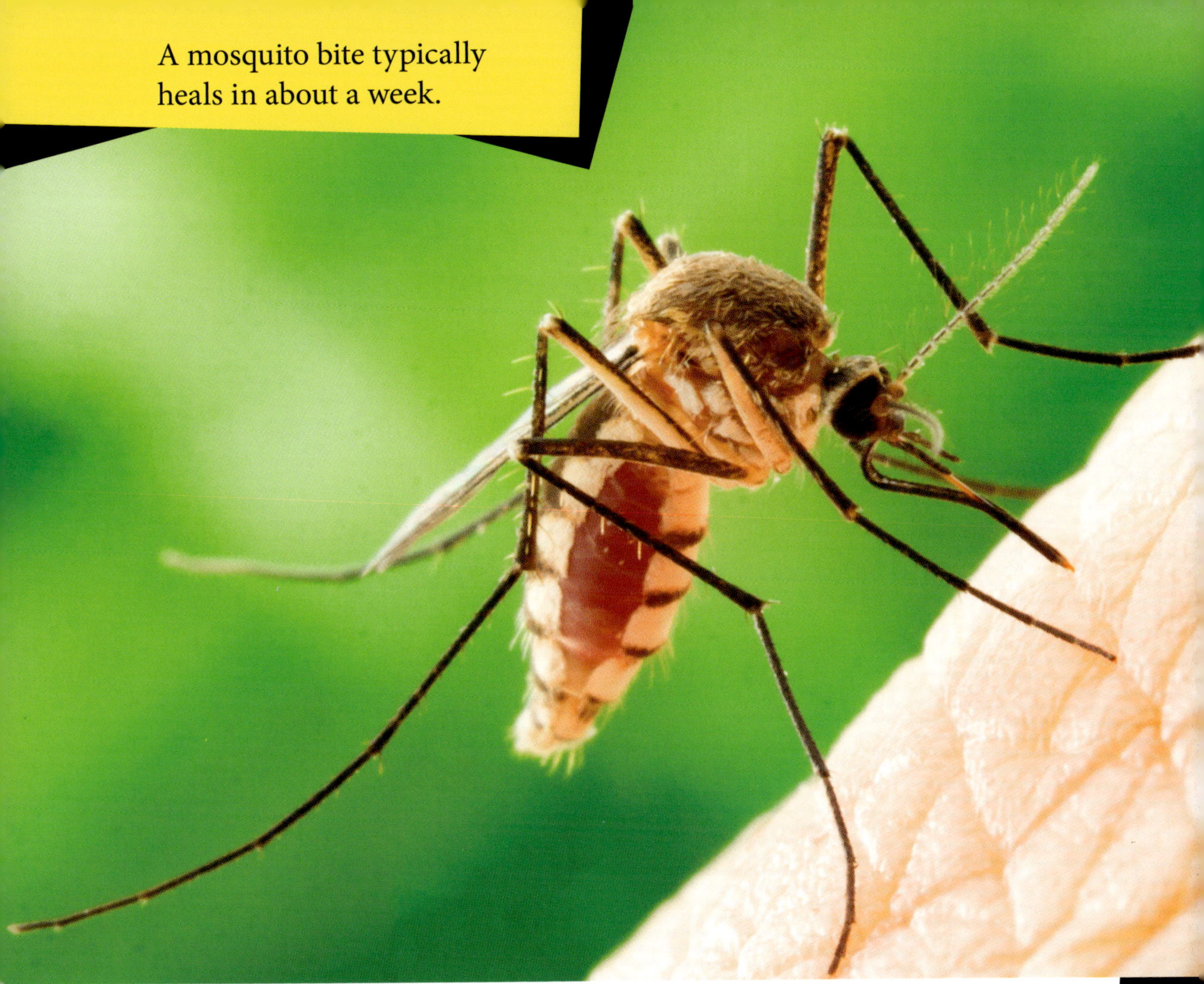

A mosquito bite typically heals in about a week.

THE DEADLY MOSQUITO

Mosquitoes carry the roundworm larvae that cause elephantiasis. They also carry malaria, yellow fever, and other diseases. Each year, about 725,000 people die from mosquito-carried diseases. That makes mosquitoes the world's deadliest animal.

GLOSSARY

acupuncture (AK-yoo-pungk-chur)—a way of treating illness by pricking parts of the body with small needles

cryogenics (kry-uh-JEN-iks)—the process of quickly freezing dead bodies in the hopes of bringing them back to life

diabetes (dy-uh-BEE-teez)—a disease in which there is too much sugar in the blood

hormone (HOR-mohn)—a chemical that affects development

host (HOHST)—a living thing from which another gets food

larva (LAR-vuh)—an insect stage between an egg and an adult

lymph (LIMF)—a clear liquid that carries nourishment and oxygen to body cells and carries away waste products

paralysis (puh-RAL-uh-siss)—a loss of the power to move or feel

parasite (PAIR-uh-site)—an animal or plant that lives on or inside another animal or plant and causes harm

phobia (FOH-bee-uh)—extremely strong fear of something

tapeworm (TAYP-wurm)—a long, flat parasite

toxin (TOK-sin)—a poison produced by a living thing

transplant (TRANSS-plant)— an operation in which a diseased organ is replaced with a healthy one

READ MORE

Bennett, Howard J. *The Fantastic Body: What Makes You Tick & How You Get Sick*. Emmaus, PA: Rodale Kids, 2017.

Biskup, Agnieszka. *Medical Marvels: The Next 100 Years of Medicine.* North Mankato, MN: Capstone Press, a Capstone imprint, 2017.

Price, Sean Stewart. *The World's Deadliest Animals.* North Mankato, MN: Capstone Publishing, 2017.

INTERNET SITES

KidsHealth from Nemours
kidshealth.org/en/kids/?WT.ac=p2k

National Geographic Kids: Wacky Weekend: Deadly Animals,
kids.nationalgeographic.com/explore/wacky-weekend/deadly-creatures/

Science for Kids: Human Body Facts
www.scienceforkidsclub.com/human-body.html

INDEX